BOUNDARIES
FOR WOMEN PHYSICIANS

Paperback ISBN 979-8-9855534-1-3
Ebook IBSN 979-8-9855534-0-6
Hardback ISBN 979-8-9855534-2-0
Audiobook ISBN 979-8-9855534-3-7

BOUNDARIES
FOR WOMEN PHYSICIANS

Love Your Life
and Career
in Medicine

TAMMIE CHANG, MD

I commend Dr. Tammie Chang for her commitment to empower women in medicine who are under so much added stress now. We need our woman physicians to be strong, happy and fulfilled. Boundaries are a key skill for them to achieve this, and Dr. Chang can help. She is a wonderful, warm teacher.

JUDITH ORLOFF, MD
New York Times Bestselling Author, The Empath's Survival Guide

Where was this book when I needed it 10 years ago? This is a book that is going to save the lives and sanity of thousands of women physicians. It is well researched and addresses the burnout epidemic in medicine. However, it also is chockful of great insight and practical tools to establish Boundaries, absolutely an essential (and dare I say, the bedrock) strategy to beat burnout. Dr. Tammie skillfully guides her reader through their journey from Burnout to Being joyous and fulfilled in medicine. This book is a must read for all female physicians. From medical students to attendings.
      Truly life changing!!!

YASHODA BHASKAR, MD
Internal Medicine, Certified Life and Money Coach

Boundaries for Women Physicians is a reminder for every female physician that she is the architect of her life. It is a blueprint for taking back control and leveraging the personal power within to build a career in medicine that is fulfilling. Read it and share a copy with your doctor sister-friend because our collective power is unstoppable!

TERRI MALCOLM, MD, MBA, CPE, ACC
CEO of Master Physician Leaders and Physician Executive Coach

As a young female physician, no one told me the dirty little secret that, in order to thrive (and even survive) in practice, it is imperative to lose those "good student" habits and resist the natural inclination to always go above and beyond at the expense of my own wellbeing (as both practices were cultivated and rewarded through my many years of school and medical training), but here Tammie makes it clear that these changes are nonnegotiable. I can hear Tammie cheering me on through the text with her friendly but firm urging because she wants better for me. Not only does she offer clear demonstrations of the consequences of lack of boundaries via the stories of relatable, well-intentioned women physicians, but she also shares practical solutions for prioritizing self-care and boundary-setting in your own life in a step-by-step fashion through reflection, promoting each of us to release some of the burdens we carry so that we have the space to grow into the best versions of ourselves.
      I am grateful for the strong, caring, bold women physicians ahead of me, like Tammie, who are trailblazers, carving a path for a brighter, kinder, more sustainable culture in medicine for generations of women physicians to come. I've already thought of countless other brilliant, dedicated, thoughtful women physician colleagues (and dear friends) who can benefit from the secrets within these pages and I can't wait to share this book with them!

BRITTANY COWFER, MD
Pediatric Hematology/Oncology

This is the most comprehensive book on boundaries for physicians. Dr. Chang provides the perfect balance of scientific evidence, personal experience and real-world action steps that will leave you feeling empowered, inspired and motivated to take action.

KRISTIN YATES, DO
Obstetrics/Gynecology, Coach

The first aid kit for today's modern women physicians: Dr. Chang provides compassionate and practical advice that can be put into practice stat.

DAVID ROSS GOSHORN, MD
Pediatric Hematology/Oncology

Healthy boundaries are absolutely crucial to our mental and emotional health as well as to our success as physicians. Yet all too often as women, we were not taught and sometimes even actively discouraged from learning and implementing this vital life skill. This book provides an amazing foundation for that, guiding the reader all the way from reframing boundaries in a positive perspective to building and then enforcing those boundaries in our personal and professional lives. It's a truly amazing resource that I can't recommend enough!

KELLY MANN, MD
Pediatric Infectious Disease

Boundaries for Women Physicians is a compelling, thought-provoking book filled with both high-level concepts and practical tips aimed specifically at women physicians. For any female doctors grappling with burnout, this book is vital and could be the beginning of a journey leading back to the joy and fulfillment we all experienced when we started our careers in medicine. And even for those who aren't worried about burnout, this book offers ideas many of us have never considered but should. This book is well worth reading and reflecting on, and I highly recommend it for all women physicians!

JENNIFER BARKLEY, MD
Internal Medicine-Pediatrics

Boundaries for Women Physicians is engaging, informative, and actionable. Well-defined boundaries in all areas of life are at the core of how we can best thrive. As one of us, Dr. Tammie Chang truly understands the demands placed on women physicians. She starts with relatable personal stories illustrating how a lack of boundaries can lead to burnout. This is followed by step-by-step actions we can take to start saying yes to ourselves. I think all women physicians will find a pearl or two in this high yield book. While succinct, it still creates space for us to reflect on own thoughts. I highly recommend it for anyone looking to start taking things off their plate so they can have the space to breathe and just be.

CHERIE CHU, MD
Pediatrics, Founder - Doctor Mom's Lounge and Wellness Pediatrician

Now more than ever it's absolutely essential for physicians to be intentional in creating their ideal lives both in and out of medicine. I absolutely believe this will make for happier physicians, better care for patients, and ultimately a better society. Dr. Chang is an amazing example of what's possible and has created a resource that we can all benefit from.

PETER KIM, MD
Anesthesiology, Founder - Passive Income MD

This book not only shows us how to build the critical skill of self-compassion into our lives, but it will also deepen our compassion for our colleagues, mentees and patients. It's a win-win-win. This book should be gifted to every graduating woman medical student. As a physician who experienced burn out herself, I only wish I had this book during those formative years.

OLGA LEMBERG, MD
Pediatrics, Founder - Fabled

Dr. Chang has put together a fantastic self-help book for women physicians who are suffering from burnout with easy-to-understand solutions to the problems that are commonly known but often not addressed. She focuses on the subject that many women deal with given our multiple roles in society: boundary setting. To make it more valuable to the reader, she divides the topics of boundaries into sections based on issues not just about ones we may deal with at work and home but also about ones we may experience in our own minds. There are many case examples that women may identify with which allow women physicians to better identify with the lives of other women physicians just like them and poignant, targeted questions that the reader is asked to answer to help them uncover the solutions. Without asking ourselves the critical questions, we may never be able to create the solutions.

Although this book is relevant to women physicians at any stage of their career, I especially like this for the early-career physicians who may not even have heard about the concept of setting boundaries. Thank you Dr. Chang for writing this book! I love seeing physicians supporting other physicians, and especially women physicians helping other women physicians.

ELSIE KOH, MD MHL
CEO and Founder of LEAD Physician® Leadership Program

Women physicians at any career stage will find resonant reflections of themselves in Dr. Chang's candid exploration of burnout and recovery. Swimming against the traditional cultures of medicine and gender, Dr. Chang makes a bold argument for the importance of focusing our immense intellectual, emotional and spiritual resources on the most unlikely of recipients: ourselves. This book is a tangible and accessible roadmap for a potentially life-saving career transformation that's not just sustainable but energizing and fulfilling.

ROBYN ROGERS, MD
Pediatric Hospital Medicine

Dr. Chang's book on boundaries was shockingly fun to read and work through. Her physician examples really hit home. I felt like she was describing me or my closest friends in our daily struggles! The worksheets are a great way to break down and work on issues in small bits. I expect to read and reread this book to deepen my practice of setting my personal boundaries.

SARA AHMED, MD
Pediatric Emergency Medicine

Boundaries for Women Physicians is the type of book we need for the 21st century woman physician. Because of her experience as a formerly burned out physician and a current physician coach, Tammie Chang brings the warmth, familiarity and hard truths necessary for women in medicine to feel empowered to design lives they genuinely enjoy and don't simply tolerate. This book has a wonderful mix of practical guidance and reflection prompts for anyone looking to make the most of her life inside and outside of work."

JATTU SENESIE MD FACOG
Physician Satisfaction Specialist/Coach/Speaker, Founder - Essence of Strength

In *Boundaries for Women Physicians*, Dr Tammie Change reveals her life experience: "I rarely slept more than four hours a night" and there were "thoughts in my head that I couldn't possibly keep going at this pace forever... But I didn't know any other way to be." This led to a low-low point of "I can't do it anymore." Sound familiar?

Thank goodness, she figured it out and is sharing how with all of us! Every physician can find themselves in the 3 scenarios in this book and benefit from creating boundaries.

You too can reach a place like Tammie where she proclaims "I love my life now. I am in the best shape physically, mentally, and emotionally of my life. I am flourishing...I feel deeply alive." I had several "ah-ha" moments when reading this book and realize I have the power to make changes in my life by setting boundaries. You can too!

MARION MCCRARY, MD
Physician Coach and Well-Being Champion, Co-Creator ResetMD Podcast

This book is a must read for any woman physician starting in their first job, as well as any struggling further in her career. It's full of practice advice for surviving that your attendings never told you during training. The imagery and examples help immerse you in a better world you can imagine for yourself. Then, the book gives you journaling prompts and thought-provoking questions to help you do the work to improve your life and grow as a woman physician. It's a perfectly balanced toolbox of low hanging fruit (do your notes really need to be that detailed?) and tough questions to help you reflect and thrive in your career and life in general. Highly recommend!

VANESSA TOLBERT, MD
Pediatric Hematology/Oncology

Dr. Tammie Chang's latest book is an exceptional read! No matter where you practice or what you do, her personal stories will resonate with you and touch your soul. It's positive words and affirmations inspired me to take control of my life and live the life I have always imagined.

JAMIE FLERLAGE, MD
Pediatric Hematology/Oncology

A MUST read for ALL women physicians!! Creating boundaries and confidently protecting them is a life-saving skill and this book gently guides you with important reflections, vivid examples and doable strategies on how to set and protect boundaries for yourself. Dr. Tammie Chang courageously shares how her life and the lives of other women physicians are saved because of boundaries!

LUISA DURAN, MD
Endocrinology, Co-Founder of Pink Coat, MD

We learn so much in our medical training, but it wasn't until I met Tammie that I realized how much I hadn't learned about myself. Defining my boundaries in my personal re-education has allowed me to become a better person and physician.

AMANDA LARSON, MD
Pediatric Orthopedic Surgery

Tammie has exceptional insight into the conflicts, challenges, and wonders women physicians experience. She gets to the root of our passions, disappointments, and stressors, and makes us realize we have the power to be fulfilled professionally and personally. Her encouragement of our taking care of ourselves first creates support, self-love and strength, allowing happiness and fulfillment in our hearts and homes.

DANA CHORTKOFF, MD
Obstetrics-Gynecology

Tammie Chang's book is a must read for all women who are practicing medicine! It is a thoughtfully written, concise, heartfelt and honest look at the ups and downs of being a woman in medical practice. It helps the reader understand the importance of setting boundaries and prioritizing one's personal needs. I wish that this been book had been around when I was starting my career!

JOAN BURG, MD
Emergency Medicine

A relatable, heartwarming and practical guide to living a full and satisfying life as a woman physician. Tammie outlines the power of boundaries in caring for ourselves and learning to thrive.

ANNIE MCCABE, MD
Pediatric Hospital Medicine

Tammie's writing and teaching on boundaries Is relatable and easy to read. It is incredibly important for us as physicians who often put everyone else ahead of us to define our boundaries to preserve our physical and mental health, which in turn will have positive effects on our relationships with family, friends and colleagues and help us provide top notch care to our patients. Once we have started to tackle boundaries, we can become examples and advocates for those around us to do the same.

SARAH WALKER, MD
Pediatric Surgery

This book is full of wonderful insight from a fellow woman doctor who has been at rock bottom but who found her way to thriving without leaving medicine. Dr. Tamara Chang guides you with actionable steps on how to set your own personal and professional boundaries to have the life and career you desire. Just about every woman doctor struggles with boundaries and this book will help you understand why they are so important.

ARCHANA SHRESTHA, MD
CoFounder and Chief Wellness Officer of Women in White Coats

In Dr. Tammie Chang's book *Boundaries for Women Physicians* she brings important data driven concepts to the table that demand our attention. Dr. Chang not only illuminates some of the difficult to discuss problems in our culture of healthcare she provides real-time solutions that work!

The facts are this: physicians are dying by suicide and leaving their jobs at alarming rates. This is a public health crisis; one that we cannot afford to ignore any longer.

Our training nor our fields address the complexities of how to create and enjoy a happy and successful life as a surgeon. It's not because we don't care; we are simply unaware of the gaps in knowledge and skills required. Reading this book is an important beginning for all of us as we consider our values, our WHY, our impact.

I am no expert. I am learning what my boundaries are, how to hold them in place, and what self-compassion even means. What I do know is that I have countless mentees who are interested in medicine and even surgery, and I want all of us to not only be successful but also for all of us to be happy in our chosen fields. This book gives me hope for our profession.

I love the advice and the self-work that is included. Do yourself a favor and make the time to follow the workbook! I love how Dr. Chang walks the reader through difficult emotions. This book made me cry and gives me hope.

ELIZABETH BERDAN, MD, MS
Pediatric General & Thoracic Surgeon

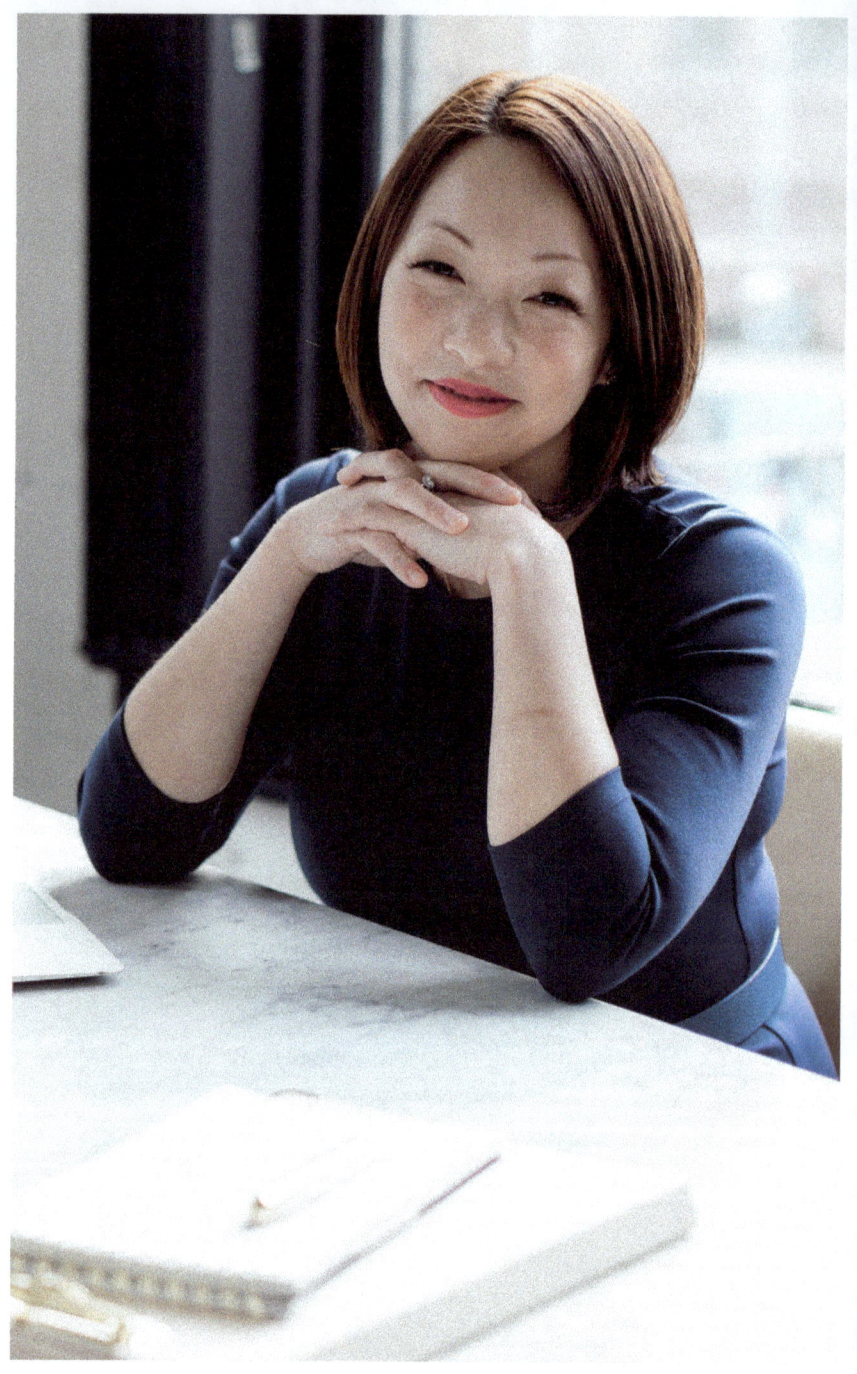

For all current and future women in medicine,
May you recognize your inherent wisdom and strength.
May you inspire others to follow your lead.

SOME GIFTS
FOR MY READERS

Enjoy!

Gift #1
Boundaries and Burnout Meter Quiz

Gift #2
Boundaries for Women Physicians
Companion Workbook

Gift #3
Boundaries Journal

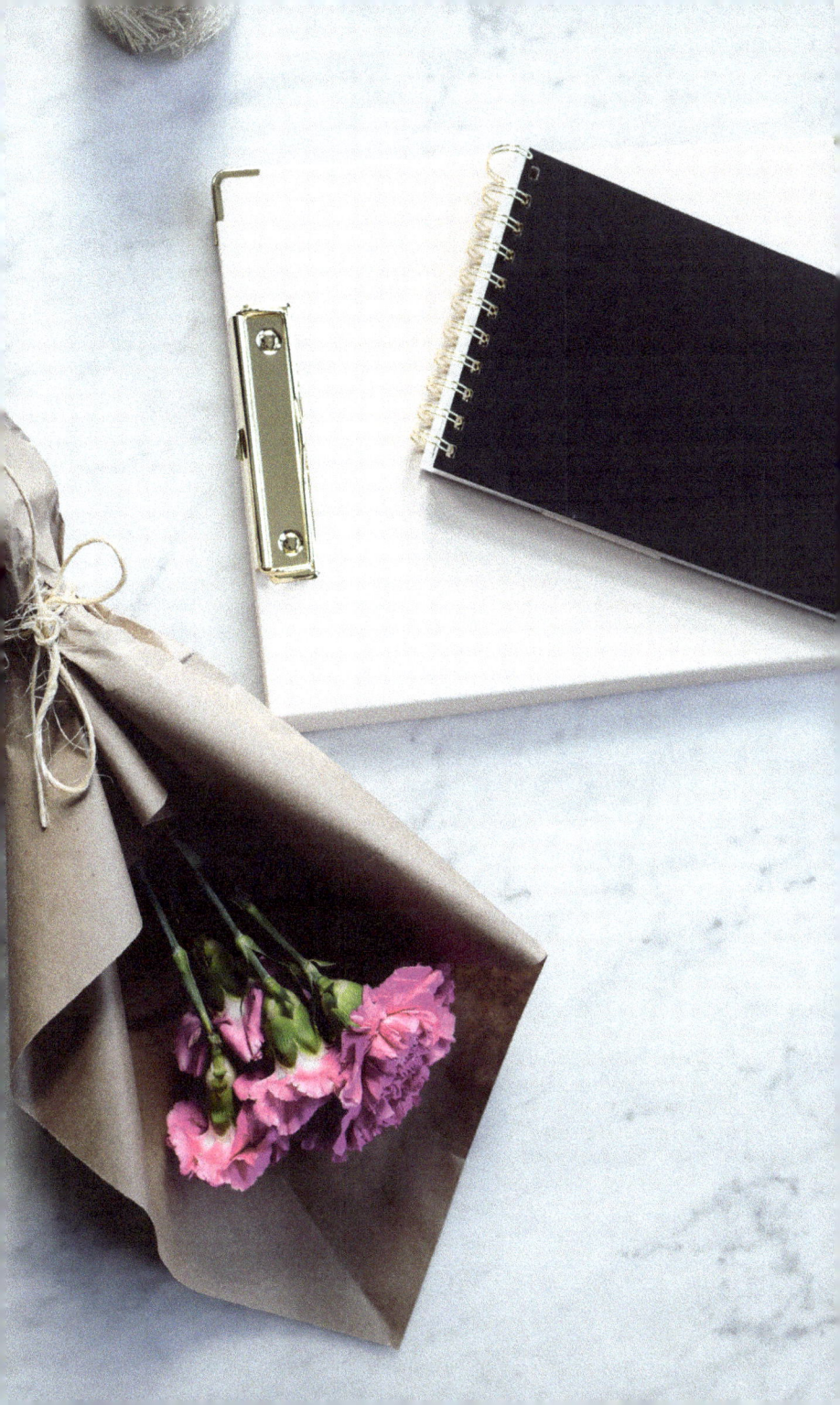

CONTENTS

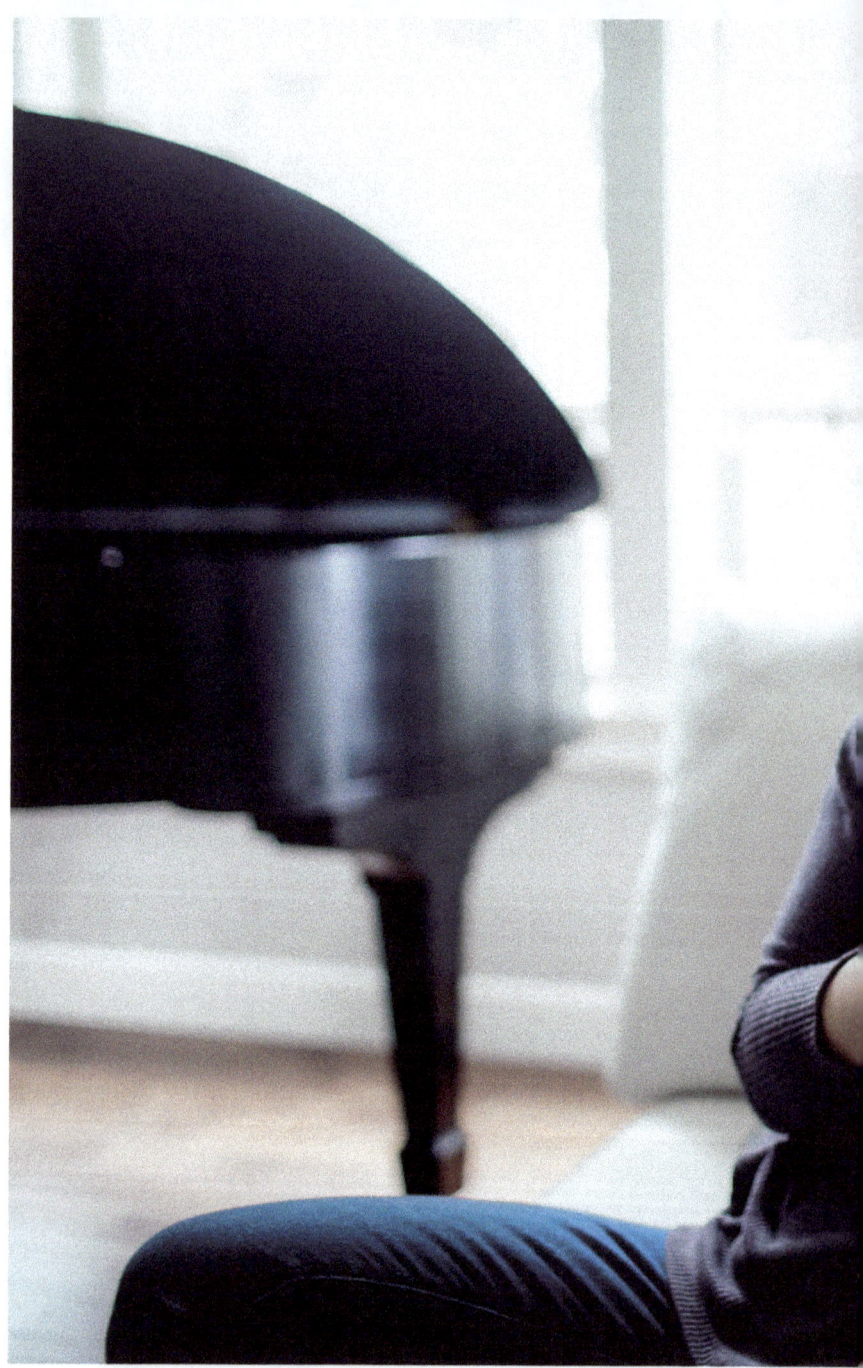

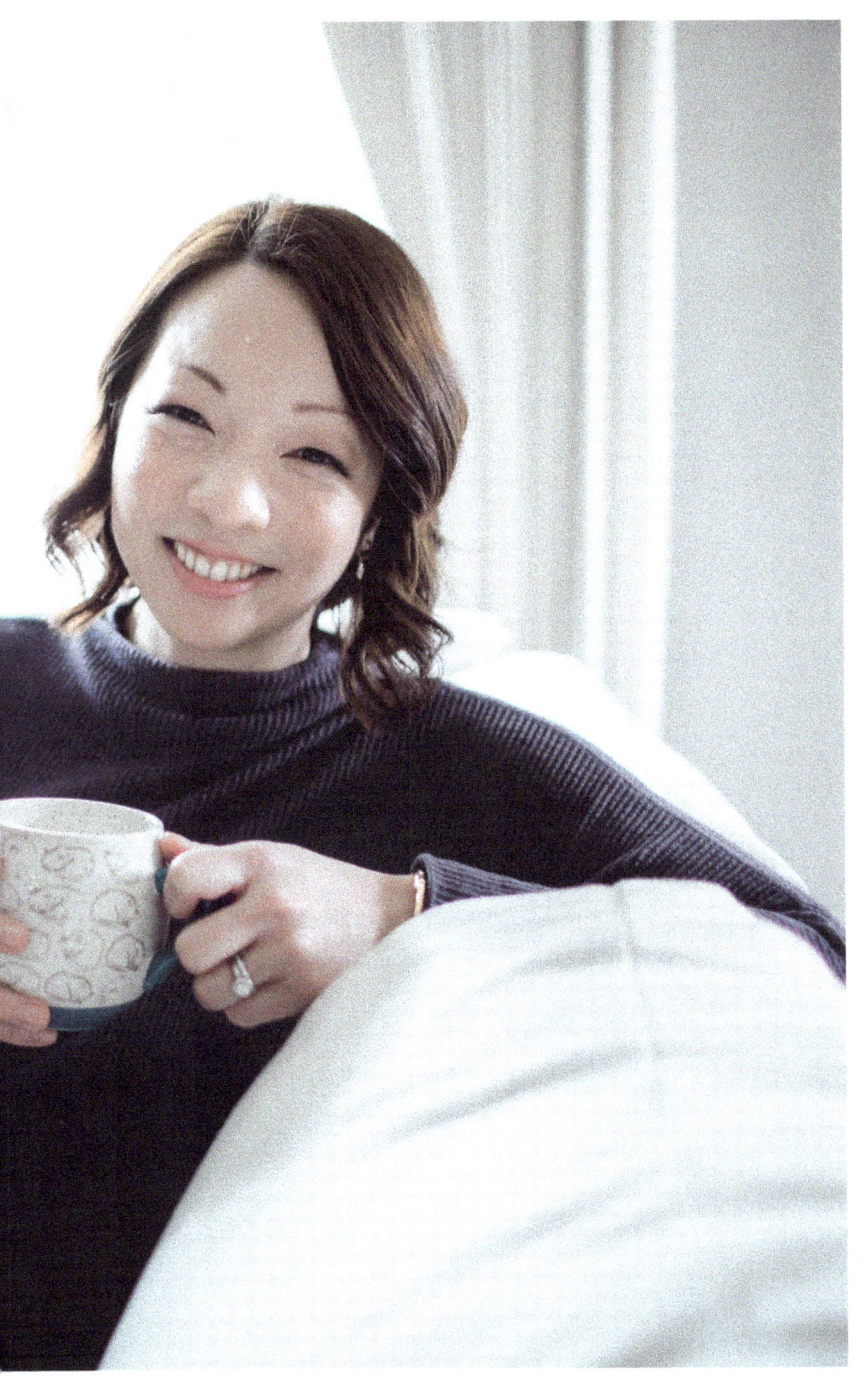

INTRODUCTION

WATCH VIDEO MESSAGE
FROM TAMMIE

My Story

My story is similar to that of countless other women who have chosen careers in medicine. I am a pediatric hematologist/oncologist. A few years ago, I was driving home one afternoon after having spent several hours with a family while they made the difficult decision to withdraw care from their terminally ill daughter. After two years of caring for them and their daughter, the tumor had come back and continued to grow, despite every type of available therapy. Their daughter had spent the last several months in the hospital. And finally, when she was no longer conscious, we knew the end had come.

At these crisis moments, I usually feel deeply connected to my patients and their families and completely in tune with my calling to serve others. While intense and emotionally draining, these times are typically when I am at my best as a physician, when I am most in possession of my inner power and wisdom, and when I feel most vital. However, that day as I was leaving the hospital, I felt exhausted in every way: emotionally, physically, mentally, and spiritually.

For months, our team had been understaffed and reeling with the responsibility of caring for record numbers of new pediatric oncology diagnoses, relapses, and deaths. Added to that had been the deaths of family members, including the young daughter of one of my colleagues. I felt responsible for the well-being of everyone in my group and went above and beyond to help them deal with all of their difficulties. I hadn't slept well in weeks and had worked every other week and weekend on call for months. I'd gained twenty pounds and couldn't remember when I'd last had time to exercise, eat a healthy meal, or connect with my husband.

As I drove home that afternoon, the idea of having to return to work at the hospital the next day was unbearable. I kept thinking, "I can't do this anymore." I imagined ways to hurt myself so that I would become incapacitated and unable to work. Rounding a curve, I experienced the strong urge to drive off the cliff. Stunned, I pulled over and sat in my car, frozen for what felt like an eternity. I was numb—too numb to cry or to feel any emotion.

When I finally made it home, I immediately called my closest friend, the one who knows me like family. He said, "Tammie, it's time for you to put on your big girl pants. You know how to have hard conversations; you do it all the time with patients and families. And now you have to do it for yourself."

So, I called my boss and said, "I can't do this anymore. I need help." I felt guilty, knowing that my sudden absence would be a tremendous burden on my colleagues. But I simply couldn't work. I needed to take a break to take care of myself.

This low point became the most important learning experience of my life.

During my leave of absence, I not only got help—a lot of it—but gained valuable perspective on the difficult working conditions for many physicians—especially women physicians, who are disproportionately affected by emotional exhaustion, burnout, and suicide; are poorly represented in leadership; and often feel compelled to switch to part-time work or leave the workforce altogether due to societal pressures. While away from work, I also discovered the value of coaching, and became a coach myself, going through multiple highly respected coaching certifications.

I came back from my leave of absence on fire to change our culture of medicine to make things better for doctors. To do this, I not only returned to my work as a pediatric hematologist/oncologist but also took on several new roles. I became the Medical Director of Provider Wellness for my large healthcare system, tasked with creating a culture of well-being for our 4,000 providers. And with one of my Brown Medical School classmates, I co-founded Pink Coat, MD, a large digital community and platform designed to bring easily accessible, high-quality, evidence-based resources and professional coaching to women physicians to help them thrive in their lives and careers. I also founded a flourishing coaching business that serves early-career women physicians who want to rise into leadership. And I co-founded ELEVATE, the American Medical Women's Associations' first leadership development program for women physicians.

My low point forced me to examine my life as a doctor and to formulate my personal mission: to improve the culture for women in medicine now, and for future generations.

Why I Wrote This Book

I learned the hard way what can happen when physicians—especially women physicians—lack personal boundaries. Before hitting my low point, I had no boundaries. I had been raised to give, give, give, and, when times became tough, to give more by working harder. In medical school and training, we were taught to not have boundaries, but rather to do everything in the service of our patients who should always come first. Now I realize that we physicians must put ourselves first. We are hurting ourselves—and doing a disservice to our patients, colleagues, and families—when we put everyone and everything else before our own needs. After all, we are our most precious resource and must use that resource in the best way possible.

As physicians and as women, we experience the double whammy of intense professional and societal expectations. As physicians, we are to care for our patients, staff, and colleagues. And then as women, it is assumed we will also tend to our children, parents, partners, friends, and neighbors. Some of us might even experience a triple whammy of expectations with additional responsibilities dictated to us by our heritage. I am one of them. As a first-generation, first-born, Asian female, I was born into many expectations in addition to those of being a woman physician.

In short, women are often expected to do the impossible: to be everything to everyone. But until we realize this is impossible, we try courageously to fulfill all these roles, and we exhaust ourselves in the process. Eventually, we find that we have nothing left to give to anyone. Nothing.

When I speak with other women physicians about maintaining boundaries, the one commonality I hear is their visceral rejection of the concept. They understand the need to establish a boundary in the first place, protecting themselves by telling others, "Don't cross this line." However, these statements are immediately followed by, "Maintaining this boundary makes me feel guilty and selfish. I am not supposed to be selfish, so I should give in." Why is holding to our boundaries so difficult for us? Why do we feel guilty and selfish when we are simply protecting ourselves and our lives? We'll explore these questions in this book.

For now, let's turn the concept of "boundaries" on its side and look at it differently. The simple truth of boundaries is that they enable us to protect our most precious resource—our life energy—so we are free to be the healers, partners, parents, friends, and daughters we want to be. Boundaries help us to create freedom because boundaries free our souls.

You must determine where you want to use your energy to live your life to its most fulfilled potential. And you must establish boundaries to protect your life energy for this purpose. The boundaries you need are completely personal, and, deep inside, you know what they are. I'm here to walk with you as you figure out your boundaries. Together, we can do this.

My wish is for you to establish boundaries to create personal and emotional sacred space for yourself. Because from this place of strength, you will be able to create anything, including a life and a career you love as a woman in medicine. And my deepest wish is that you will then share your wisdom with every woman you know at any stage of life. When we collectively break down what holds us back as women and physicians, we create a profession full of brilliant, compassionate, and caring people. Our world improves tremendously when women like you are leading and caring for our patients, families, and communities, and I know without a doubt, the ripple effect and impact on our world will be endless.

How This Book Will Help You

What do you long to have more of in your life? What do you need less of? What boundaries do you need to create to obtain these objectives? In what areas of your life do you need assistance? Who can you ask for this assistance? In *Boundaries for Women Physicians*, we will explore these questions and then create a plan for you to achieve the life you crave. Throughout the book, I will share my own story and the stories of three hypothetical physicians to illustrate how you can create boundaries in all aspects of your life.

In Part I of this book, we will examine why boundaries are necessary. We will look at some startling statistics about our world of medicine and discuss how our medical training failed to teach us how to adequately take care of ourselves. Then we'll explore how boundaries can help us turn things around so we can begin to live the life we crave.

In Part II, we will look at why boundaries must start with us, how we must begin from a place of clarity and self-awareness to create the boundaries needed to thrive in all aspects of our lives. Because contrary to what we may believe or have been taught, to set boundaries we must begin with ourselves.

In Part III, we will continue by exploring boundaries at work, covering many of the key stressors that plague us in our workday as physicians: professional patient-physician boundaries, Electronic Medical Records (EMR), charting, colleagues, staff, and the realities of a physician's work life in today's imperfect healthcare landscape.

We will explore boundaries at home in Part IV of this book, discussing many key areas that professional women—especially women physicians—struggle with, such as multiple roles, family, friends, children, our homes, money, and carving out a physical and emotional space for ourselves.

Lastly, in Part V we will put all of this together as I walk you through a step-by-step process to creating your customized Whole-Life Boundary Plan.

Your Boundaries Journal

For you to get the most out of this book, I suggest you buy a special notebook to use as your Boundaries Journal. Use it to jot down any information you find particularly relevant to your life, and to record your answers to the reflection questions at the end of each chapter, which are designed to help you explore key ideas.

When you see this gold box and symbol, this signifies a reflective journaling exercise.

Boundaries Workbook

In addition, I have created a workbook containing the worksheets for the exercises in this book. Using the QR code or hyperlink found at the beginning of this book, download your copy of the workbook, now. Throughout the book, I also have included hyperlinks and QR codes for videos of additional information and encouragement.

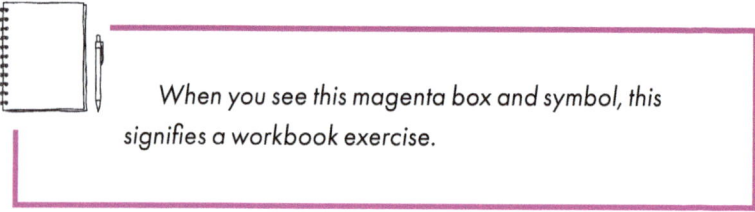

When you see this magenta box and symbol, this signifies a workbook exercise.

As you read this book, please remember I will be here as your partner and your guide every step of the way, just as I am with each of my women physician coaching clients. As a physician myself, my hunch is that you love checking things off your to-do list. With this book, you can check off "Setting My Boundaries" from your list for good.

Let's do this, friend— I've got you!

Tammie

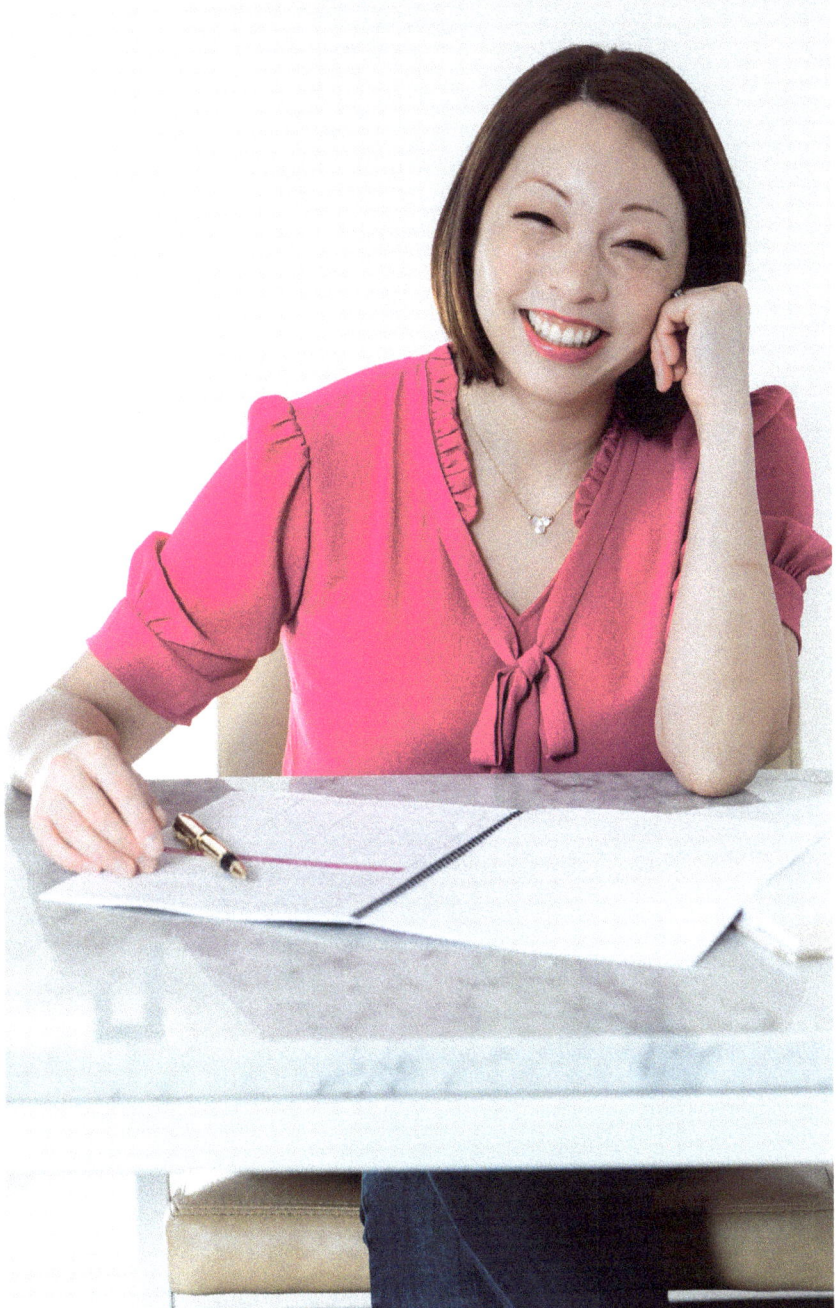

WATCH VIDEO MESSAGE
FROM TAMMIE

PART I

WHY BOUNDARIES ARE NECESSARY

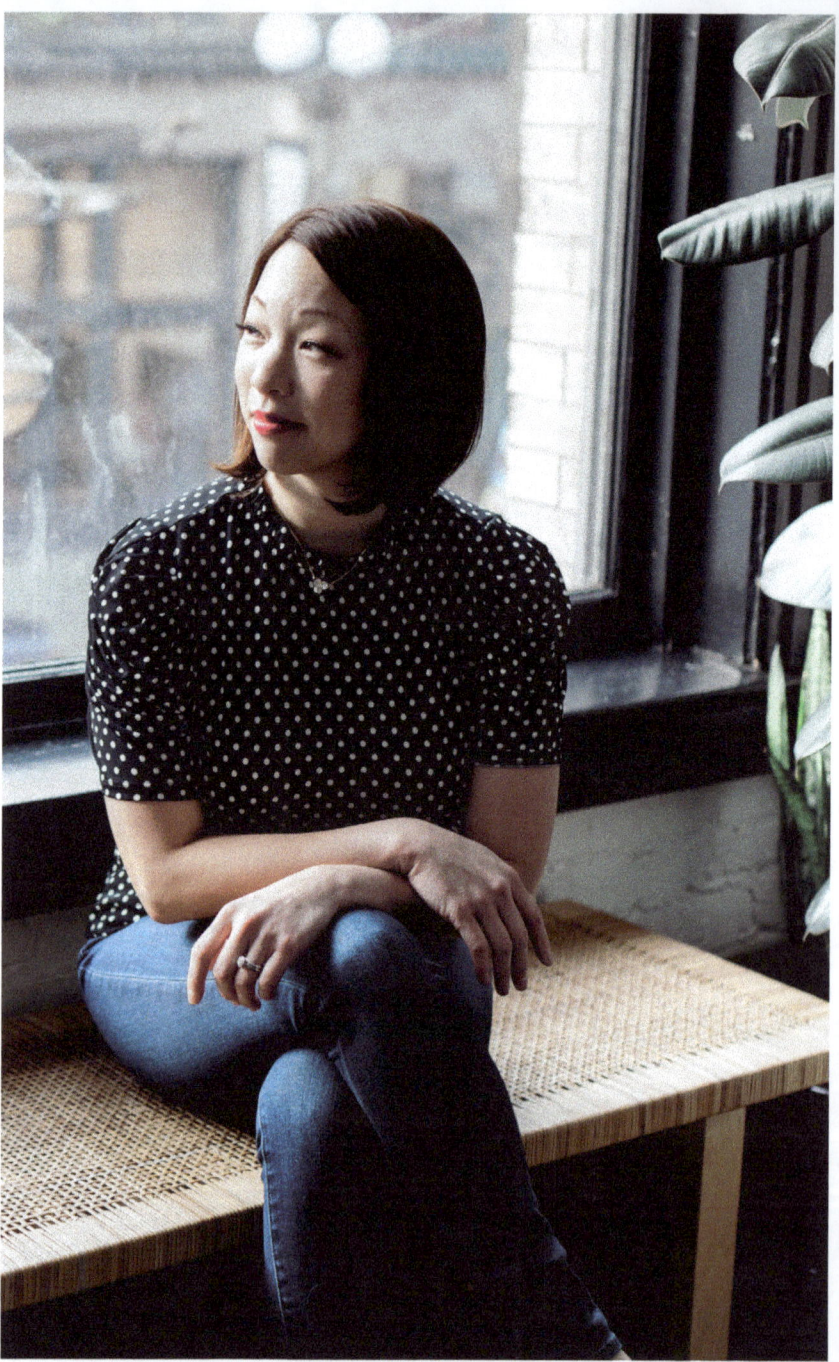

CHAPTER 1

THE REALITY:
BURNOUT, EMOTIONAL EXHAUSTION, STRESS, AND SUICIDE

Our Silent Suffering

When I openly share my experiences with friends and colleagues, I am amazed by how many other women physicians tell me they have had similar ones. They admit to feeling so low that suicide or self-harm seems the only way out. They tell me they've experienced this countless times, especially during their training. Many of them say they feel so alone, as if they're living in their own hell. My heart breaks when I hear these stories.

As I was researching this book, I learned that my experience, and that of so many others, is reflected in overwhelming data:

- Female physicians are 60% more likely to suffer from emotional exhaustion and burnout than male physicians (West et al., 2018).
- Women physicians are at as much as a 400% increased risk

of dying from suicide compared with women in the general population (Hampton, 2005).

- Women physicians are quitting medicine at alarming rates, with 40% either going part-time or quitting medicine altogether within six years of completing their residency training (Paturel, 2019).

What?!?

Even though I had been on a track to become a physician since I was 18 years old, spending 20 years immersed in medical training and culture, this was the first time I had ever heard these statistics. I wondered, why the secrecy?

The conversation we need to have about burnout, suicide, emotional exhaustion, and the mental health crisis in medicine is just now beginning. For too long our profession has made practitioners feel ashamed of their own suffering, suppressed in a centuries-old culture of silence. As physicians, we are taught not to show weakness, doubt, or vulnerability. We are told that we must be strong for our patients, families, staff, and everyone else, even if it is at the expense of our health. It seems almost heretical to admit weakness or to need help. Our medical culture glorifies overwork. It is considered a badge of honor to be the first one to arrive in the morning and the last one to leave at night. For years I have heard physicians state with pride that they worked all evening and all weekend. I too believed this was exemplary behavior and modeled it myself, until I couldn't do it anymore.

As doctors, we are used to sucking it up. We had to in order to make it through all those late nights as medical students and the exhaustion of residency and fellowship training. But sucking it up as our only coping mechanism has led us to the crisis in medicine we are experiencing today.

Fighting for Our Lives

This medical mental health crisis doesn't affect only female physicians. Physicians overall have the highest rate of suicide among all professions and have a significantly higher risk of suicide than the general population (Schernhammer and Colditz, 2004). In the United States, 300 to 400 doctors commit suicide each year, more than double the rate in the general population (Farmer, 2018). As many as one in five physicians has considered dying by suicide (Menon and Shanafelt, 2020).

Physicians are fighting for their lives. In the 2018 documentary *Do No Harm: Exposing the Hippocratic Hoax*, director Robyn Symon exposed the epidemic of physician suicide and burnout, and the dark secret that many doctors are struggling and suffering in silence. When several physicians committed suicide during the COVID-19 pandemic, the stories were widely profiled in the media—the first many had heard about the problem. Healthcare organizations all across the country are scrambling to find solutions to this mental health crisis.

Causes

Many of the underlying causes of this crisis are factors out of the practitioner's control, such as relative value units (RVU), productivity pressures, patient satisfaction scores, publication pressures, financial limitations, complicated billing codes, and the increasing requirements of electronic medical records, charting, and bureaucratic tasks. A lack of budget for support staff forces doctors to do what had been the work of medical assistants, administrative assistants, and nurses. And inadequate physician staffing can result in unsafe patient care loads and/or being forced to work additional call hours, nights, and weekends. Our healthcare system has changed rapidly and dramatically in the past two decades. Research shows that 80% of burnout is due to systemic factors (Collier, 2018) and is not caused by a lack of individual resilience and stress management on the part of physicians.

The result of this crisis is that the profession's life and legacy are in jeopardy. In a recent study, 60% of 13,500 physicians polled would not recommend pursuing a career in medicine to their children or other young people, and more than one-third reported that they would not select medicine as a career if they had to choose again (The Physicians Foundation study, 2012).

What We Can Control

In the face of a rapidly changing healthcare landscape, with so much that is out of our control, what can we do? As physicians, we have the power to change and reframe our situation much more than we realize by altering our response to adverse external pressures. No matter how overwhelming or oppressive these pressures are, no matter how powerless or small we feel, the key to our empowerment is to develop a strong sense of internal boundaries and to prioritize our self-care. If we say "no" to unreasonable demands and expectations, the perpetual cycle of systemic burnout due to our broken healthcare system and dysfunctional culture of medicine will come to an end.

We alone can do this. No one can do it for us. No one *will* do it for us. From this place of strength, we have the power to not only survive but thrive. The key to loving our lives and our careers starts with us.

Reflection Questions

1. This chapter presents some tough data about how often women in medicine suffer from emotional exhaustion, quit practice, and commit suicide. How does this data make you feel? What strikes you most about these trends?
2. This chapter also discusses why physicians feel so overwhelmed at work. What feels out of control in your own professional life? What do you wish were different?
3. We saw that the future of our medical profession is in jeopardy, with doctors recommending against entering the field. How do you feel about this?
4. What needs to change in medicine for you to be successful?
5. What needs to change for you to love your life in medicine?

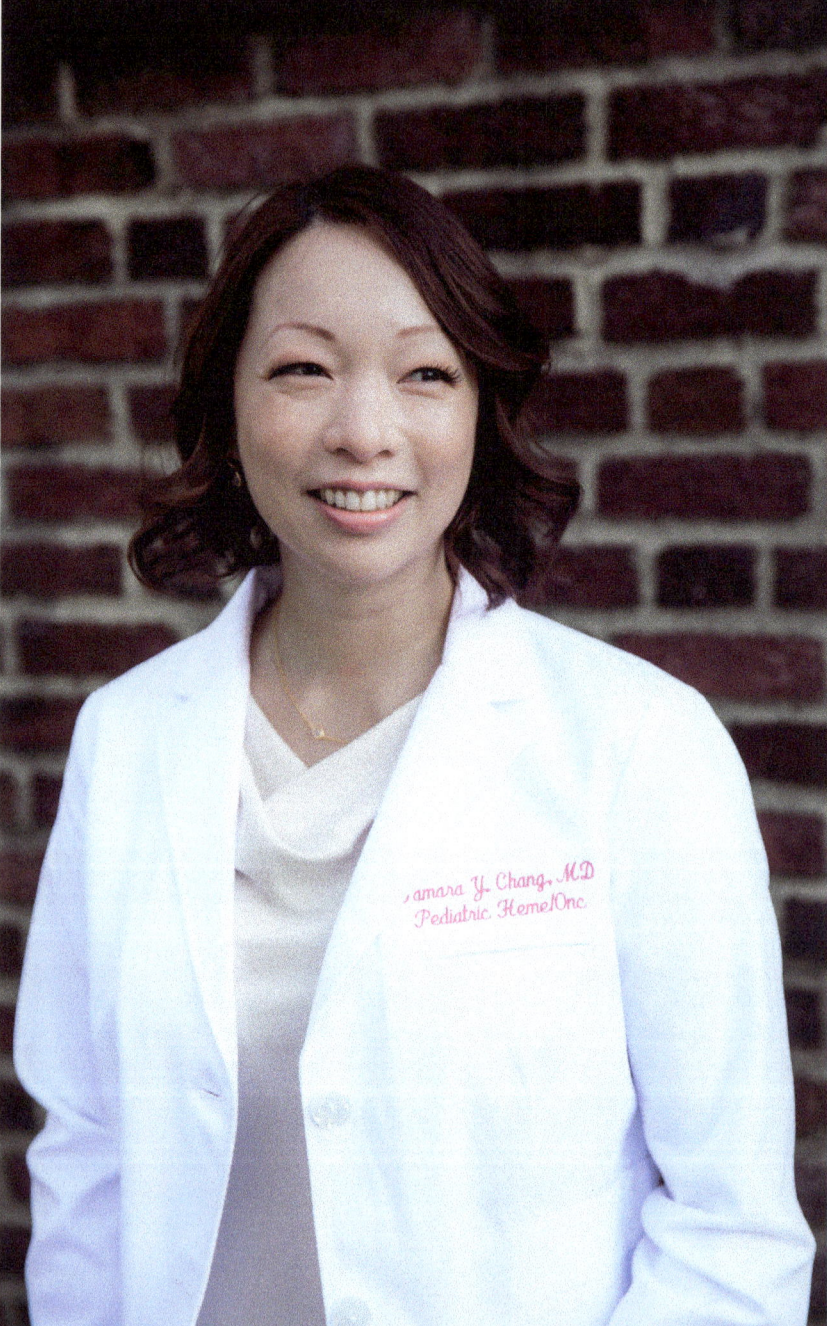

CHAPTER 2

HOW WE THINK
ABOUT BOUNDARIES

"Boundaries" is a buzzword that means different things to different people. The concept of personal boundaries didn't exist until the mid-1980s when it was introduced by therapists, self-help authors, and support groups. Personal boundaries were further popularized in the 1990s when Drs. Henry Cloud and John Townsend introduced this valuable concept in their book *Boundaries: When to Say Yes, How to Say No to Take Control of Your Life* (Zondervan, 1992). They describe our physical world as having clear boundaries in the form of fences, property lines, and even moats filled with alligators. Our personal, emotional, and spiritual boundaries are invisible to the eye, but they are just as crucial for our survival. They help us to define ourselves: what is us and what is not us, and—most importantly—what is our responsibility and what is not.

For most of us, the idea of personal boundaries was not part of our upbringing, nor was it part of our parents' upbringing. I find this perspective an important one because it sheds light on why we as women physicians struggle to set boundaries: the concept of boundaries was not taught to us or modeled for us. Therefore, we must learn how to change our behavior and attitudes about boundaries, which will take time. But if we put in the work now, one small baby step at a time, we will get there.

Boundaries as Medical Students and Trainees

As medical students, we are trained to put our patients first—above all else. We are told we are ultimately responsible for everything that happens in their care. On the wards, as naive third-year medical students, we are further indoctrinated into this culture of hyper-responsibility. We feel overly accountable to our patients, our senior residents, our attendings, the nursing staff, and everyone else. Students are praised if they come in before dawn to pre-round and stay late into the evening to ensure that everything is taken care of for their patients. They are rewarded if they work on weekends, holidays, and days off. And this continues, through internship, residency, and fellowship training.

I was one of those medical students who went the extra mile. Were you? It's no wonder that later, after years of living, breathing, and working in this world, as students, trainees, and then attendings, we struggle with setting boundaries and performing self-care.

Physicians as Human Givers

Amelia and Emily Nagoski describe Human Giver Syndrome in their book, Burnout: *The Secret to Unlocking the Stress Cycle* (Ballantine Books, 2019). According to them, human givers are expected to be "pretty, happy, calm, generous, and attentive to the needs of others" at all times. Women are socialized to exhibit such behavior much more than men. This includes the expectation that when others need us, women must be available, willing, and ready to help. If we do not comply, we are often labeled as poor team players, selfish, or not nice.

Our culture of medicine promotes the expectation that all physicians are human givers, that we go into medicine to serve our patients and put their needs before ours. And women physicians struggle with the double burden of social expectations for both women and physicians as human givers. Because of this, it's no wonder that setting and maintaining healthy boundaries seem impossible. Yet it is only after we use boundaries to protect ourselves that we can interrupt our cycle of endless giving, prioritize our own needs, and create the life we crave.

A House as a Metaphor for Our Lives

Merriam-Webster.com defines a metaphor as: "a figure of speech in which a word or phrase literally denoting one kind of object or idea is used in place of another to suggest a likeness or analogy between them." In other words, an image is used to represent a concept. This is an extremely powerful tool to use when working to affect changes in our attitudes and behaviors, because we can create a visual image of who we want to become. When discussing boundaries with women physicians, the metaphor that resonates the most is one of a well-built house surrounded by a yard and a picket fence, with the house representing us and our lives, the yard as the buffer zone between us and the outside world, and the fence as our protective boundary. Within this fence are several gates that we can choose to open or close, allowing us to decide who and what to allow into our lives, and who and what to keep out.

Visioning Exercise

Using this metaphor, imagine yourself as a house. If the outside of the house represents your physical self, what does it look like? Is it well-built and sturdy or old and broken down? Is it neat and trimmed or in need of a new paint job? Are there curtains in the windows or are they cracked and empty? What image does your house project to others?

Now, look inside your metaphorical house, with its interior representing your emotional self. What do you see? Is it welcoming and calm, with a cozy nook for reading and perhaps a kitchen full of the aroma of cinnamon bread in the oven? Do you hear the sounds of children laughing or perhaps light jazz music playing in the background? Or is your house dark and decrepit, with creaking floors, dirty windows, and a dark, scary basement? Are there rooms that you are frightened to enter and want to keep hidden from others? In general, is this house well cared for or in need of some tender loving care?

Now, look out of the front door at your yard, with the yard representing the buffer zone where you interact with others. Are neighbors and extended family members waiting on your front lawn, wanting and needing something from you? Even worse, have many of your patients and staff followed you home from work, setting up camp chairs immediately outside your door? Or is your yard filled with only the friends and family members you choose to spend your time with?

In your mind's eye, walk up to the picket fence surrounding your yard, remembering that the fence represents the boundaries you have created to protect yourself. What do you see? Is the fence in good condition: solid with fresh paint and well-built gates and latches? Or is the fence dilapidated and broken, with no latches and entire sections missing? Is the picket fence doing a good job protecting your house and yard? In other words, are your boundaries protecting you and your inner circle?

Notice how these various mental images make you feel.

Your Metaphorical House is You

You are this metaphorical house, which includes all physical, emotional, mental, and spiritual facets of yourself. As with any piece of property, you must care for this house by putting in the time, energy, and love necessary to make sure that the property is well looked after. You also must do the preventative care needed for any home by fixing the things that are beginning to break down. Caring for you—your most precious resource—is necessary to be able to be the kind of woman, physician, partner, mother, daughter, or friend you long to be.

Reflection Questions

1. We learn as young medical students to put our patients first, above all else. How have these lessons learned as a student and trainee impacted how you feel about boundaries?
2. How does the metaphor of the house resonate with you?
3. What does your house, lawn, and fence look like?
4. What parts of the house are you scared to enter? What emotion is represented by a room you didn't want to enter? What emotion is represented by a room you wanted to keep hidden?
5. As a metaphor for you and your life, what would you like your house/yard/fence to look like and feel like?

CHAPTER 3

BOUNDARIES AND
THE LIFE YOU CRAVE

In the introduction to this book, I shared how I hit rock bottom and was on the brink of suicide when a new awareness of my needs forced me to stop and finally ask for help. And then in Chapter 2, when we explored the house metaphor and mentioned having patients, parents, family members, neighbors, and work staff—essentially everyone—camped out on the front lawn, asking for something—well, that was my lawn. But this was not the fault of all these people. I realized that I alone was responsible for allowing those people to be there, and this realization led me to establish boundaries that allowed me to rebuild my life, move forward, thrive, love my work, and strive to help other women find the same freedom I have found. You might wonder, "How have boundaries done all that for you?" To understand the answer to that question, let's back up a bit.

The Drive to Serve

The need to help others was a core value instilled in me from a young age. I clearly remember the moment when it developed into a deep desire to serve. I was fifteen and heard a moving graduation speech by David Shipley '81, a former graduate of my school and a speech writer for former President Bill Clinton. "We are here to serve," were his parting words, which resonated with me at my core. I sat in the audience thinking, "Yes. That's why I am here—to help other people." For the two and a half decades since that pivotal moment in my childhood, my desire to serve others through compassion has remained my strongest motivation.

Throughout my early life, I believed my drive to serve, my sacrifice, and my relentless work ethic made me who I was and that was who I should be. I paid no attention to the fact that this altruism was almost always at the expense of my time, energy, and well-being. When I went to med school and learned the ways of our medical world, I was indoctrinated even more deeply into a culture of over-giving. I was that medical student, intern, resident, and fellow who came in on weekends and days off to check on patients, returned to the hospital on holidays to make sure they were not alone, and came back after long days on the wards to spend hours—sometimes late into the night—to sit with them and their families. This life gave me a sense of meaning and purpose. But there was no end to my giving. I did not know how to stop until there was nothing left to give.

A Life We Love

Then I learned to establish and maintain healthy boundaries and I love my life now. I am in the best physical, mental, and emotional shape of my life. I am flourishing. I love taking care of patients. I no longer feel drained by work; the needs of patients, staff, and families; or the needs of others in my life. I rarely have a backlog of unfinished chart notes, telephone messages, medication refills, or other tasks. My email inbox is finely curated. I seldom open my electronic medical records (EMR) or email between 5 p.m. and 8 a.m. or on weekends. I no longer come in on weekends or days off. I am done with my daily work and driving home by 5 p.m. When I am at home, I am at home. I have an incredible community and a group of close friends. I am more connected to family, friends, and mentors from each phase of my childhood and life than I have ever been. I am constantly learning new skills and ideas, constantly feeling challenged and stretched in the best of ways. I am creating. I have boundless energy. I am happy and full of joy. I feel deeply alive. And all of this is because I learned to set boundaries in my life.

If I can do this, I know you can, too. Boundaries are the key to creating the life you long for. Now let's do this together.

Reflection Questions

1. How will setting boundaries help you?
2. During your childhood and upbringing, what were you taught, or not taught, about boundaries? How were boundaries modeled for you? By whom?
3. What does a life of freedom look like for you?
4. What needs to change for you to love your life?

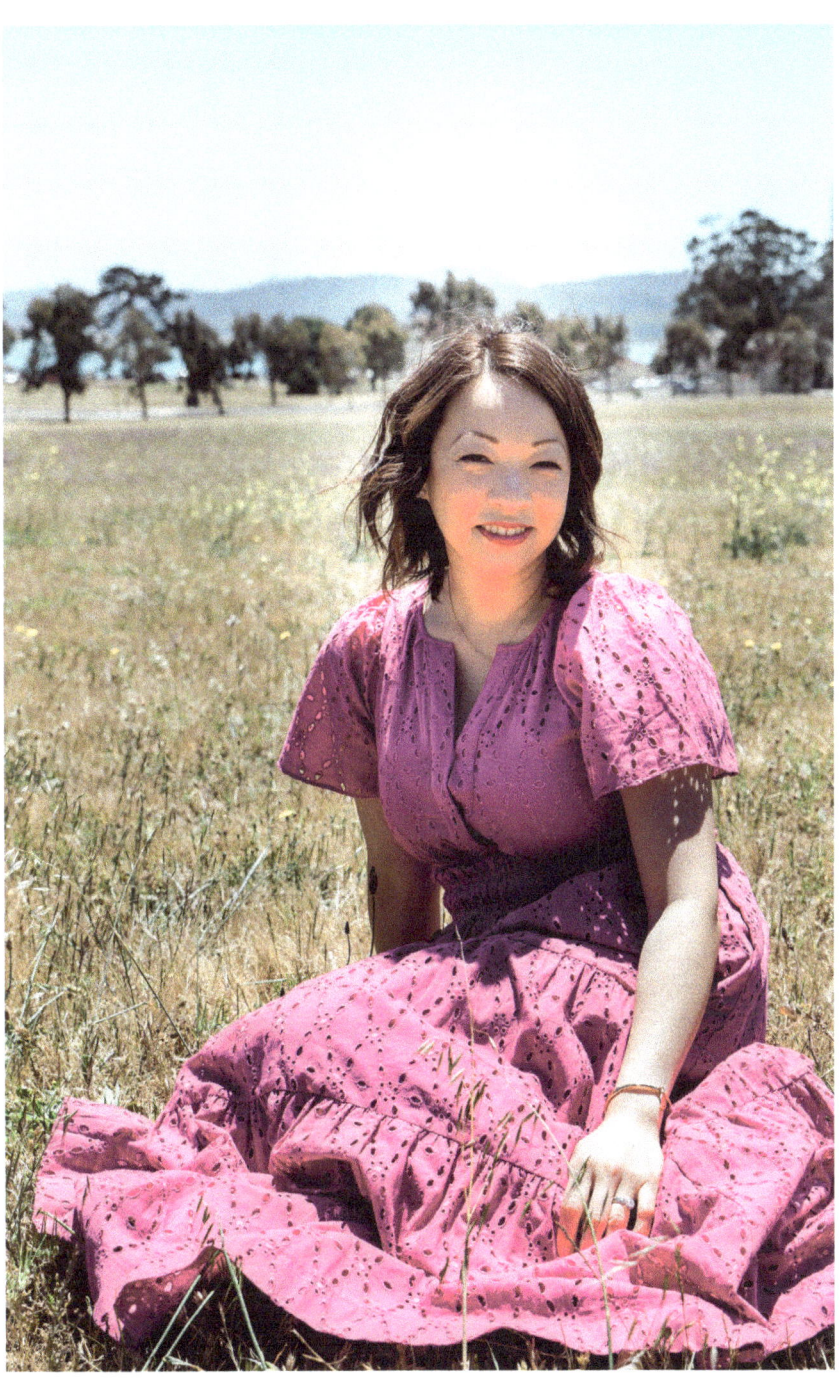

WATCH VIDEO MESSAGE
FROM TAMMIE

PART II

BOUNDARIES START WITH YOU

CHAPTER 4

KNOWING WHO YOU ARE

Meet Dr. Shruthi

Dr. Shruthi is one badass woman surgeon but does not realize this.
The oldest daughter of working-class immigrant parents and the first
person to ever attend medical school in her family, she was taught from
an early age the importance of having a strong work ethic and always
striving to do better. Medical school and residency years were tough.
As one of five women—and one of only two minority women—in her
class of 15 surgical residents, she felt she needed to prove she could be
just as good as the male surgical residents and heard this expectation
reiterated daily in her interactions with staff, attendings, and fellow
residents. Heaven forbid she ever had a bad day, felt tired, or was
hungry—no allowance was made for these normal human frailties.
There were times when she felt so exhausted, so beat down, and so low
that she sought help from a therapist. Having married a fellow doctor

during medical school, she felt her residency training severely tested their relationship. She and her husband rarely saw each other, and when they did, they were both exhausted and merely surviving. Dr. Shruthi believed she had to go through those tough, miserable years of residency training to become a surgeon, and she knew how to. She was one gritty, tough woman thanks to her parents, especially her father.

Dr. Shruthi looked forward to having a better life as an attending, and the chance to finally call her own shots. Little did she know that becoming a junior attending—and especially a junior female attending—would be harder than anything she had experienced before.

Now, two years into her life as a surgery attending at a community hospital, she is afraid there may not be an end to her life of toil and struggle. She and her husband delayed having children until after completing training. Now they desperately want to start a family but, like many of Dr. Shruthi's residency and medical school friends, find they are struggling with infertility. As a junior attending surgeon at her hospital and one of only two women surgeons, she continues to have a grueling on-call schedule, taking night calls and covering the hospital for trauma call every other weekend—significantly more hours than any of her senior male surgeon colleagues. She is scared to advocate for less time on call, as the last time a woman surgeon did this, she was labeled "a complainer" and pressured to leave the hospital. Dr. Shruthi does not want to be perceived as weak or a complainer, but she is struggling. She wants to understand who she is, what she needs, and if there could be any other kind of life for her. Having spent the last decade of her life in intense, grueling medical training, she feels overwhelmed, exhausted, and worn out. She has no hope that things will ever get better.

The Myth of Life After Training

Do you relate to Dr. Shruthi's story? I certainly do. After years of delayed gratification, spending our twenties and early thirties

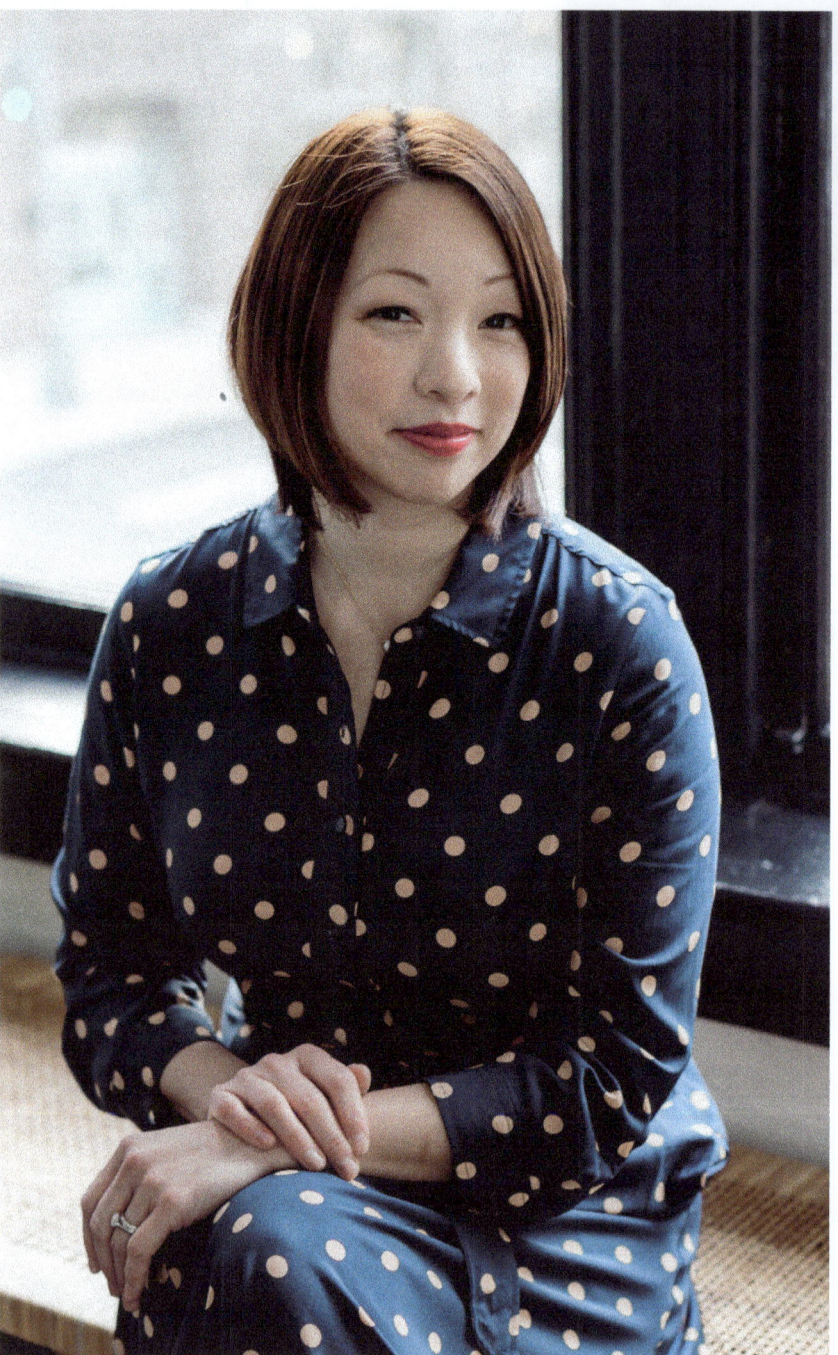

in medical training, we often emerge from those years with little awareness of our own needs, core values, priorities, or greater desires for our lives. We had to put so much on hold to just make it through. Now, having survived those years, we feel lost and overwhelmed as we realize that life after training isn't necessarily better. In fact, for many of us, it's the same or worse. We are still immersed in the same unhealthy culture of medicine: a culture espousing a relentless work ethic; unquestionable commitment to our patients, staff, and work; and the necessity of putting our personal needs last.

Taking a Meta View

Sometimes, I find it helpful to gain some perspective on my professional life by viewing it from a distance. Perhaps this might help you, too.

Imagine climbing into a hot air balloon and gently and slowly ascending into the air. Observe your life spread out below you, with its stress, toil, and hardships becoming smaller and thus easier to see and understand. When looking down at your life, what does it look like? Are there mountains, trees, valleys, rivers, streams, oceans, deserts, or cities? Are there homes, streets, neighborhoods, and kids playing on the sidewalks? What do these things represent in your life as a physician? Do you view a world of beauty, contentment, and peace? Or is it one of ugliness, pain, and anger? Is the world you see aligned with your purpose in life and what you want?

When I coach women physicians, many can articulate important themes in their lives—like the importance of family, caring for others, or service—but most struggle to succinctly articulate their life purpose and their core values. Our values and purpose are our internal compasses, our very own GPS systems, that guide us through life. They tell us who we are, what is important to us, and what is non-negotiable in our lives. When we know our life purpose and our core values, decisions and choices become easier. We may not know exactly where we are going but we have an intuitive sense that we are headed in the right direction.

We feel at peace. We are aligned with our deepest and most authentic selves.

Staying True to Ourselves as Women, Physicians, and Leaders

In her book, *Dare to Lead* (Random House, 2018), professor, TED Talk speaker, and podcast host Brené Brown explains that to be a good leader, you must stay true to your core values. As Brown writes, "A value is a way of being or believing that we hold most important. Living into our values means that we do more than profess our values, we practice them. We walk our talk—we are clear about what we believe and hold important, and we take care that our intentions, words, thoughts, and behaviors align with those beliefs." She believes the strength in leadership must come from this place of authenticity. As physicians, we are the leaders of our teams, no matter our age, experience, position, or title. Recognize that you are a leader, and thus are responsible for setting and modeling healthy values.

Our values are like our North Star; they help us to align our thoughts, behaviors, and actions with the deepest core of who we are. When we are aligned with our values, we feel more at ease and life flows more smoothly. When we are not honoring our values, we feel stressed, guilty, frustrated, or even angry. Where in your life does this show up for you?

Another valuable concept to understand is your Why—your life's purpose and how you want to uniquely contribute to the world. In his book, *Start with Why* (Portfolio, 2011), TED Talk speaker and podcast host Simon Sinek stresses the need to be in alignment with our life's purpose and emphasizes the need for leaders to begin by recognizing their purpose. "To inspire starts with the clarity of WHY," he writes. According to Sinek, when we can identify our Why, our lives are much more harmonious, we inspire others, and we have a greater impact.

So, when you are faced with a new situation, decision, or dilemma, ask yourself what choice would be most in alignment with your core values and your Why. When viewed through this lens, decisions and boundaries become clear.

Now let's discover and fine-tune your core values and your Why.

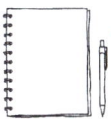

Your Core Values

When exploring your core values, think about these questions:
- What are the peak experiences in your life so far?
- When have you felt most alive?
- What makes you mad—MAD!—enough to stand up for something?
- What common themes do you notice in your life?

Now, review the list of common core values provided in your Workbook.
- Circle all the values that resonate for you.
- Then narrow this list down to your top five values.
- Rank them in order of most to least important for you.
- Place this list of your top five core values where you will see it every day, perhaps posted on your refrigerator, taped to your computer monitor, pinned to the corkboard on your wall, or pasted on the home screen of your smartphone.

Every time you are faced with making a decision, answering a question, or making a choice, look at the list of your top

...continued overleaf

core values, and ask yourself these three questions:

1. Are you honoring your core values with your answer, decision, or choice?
2. How are you not honoring your core values?
3. How could you be honoring your core values more?

Your Why

To identify your Why, consider these questions:

- What makes you want to get up in the morning?
- What do you want most in your life?
- What will having this do for you?
- How will you know when you have it?
- What impact do you want your life to have on the world?

So, friend, what is your Why? It's okay if you are not sure yet. Take time now to brainstorm some ideas in the worksheets provided in your Workbook.

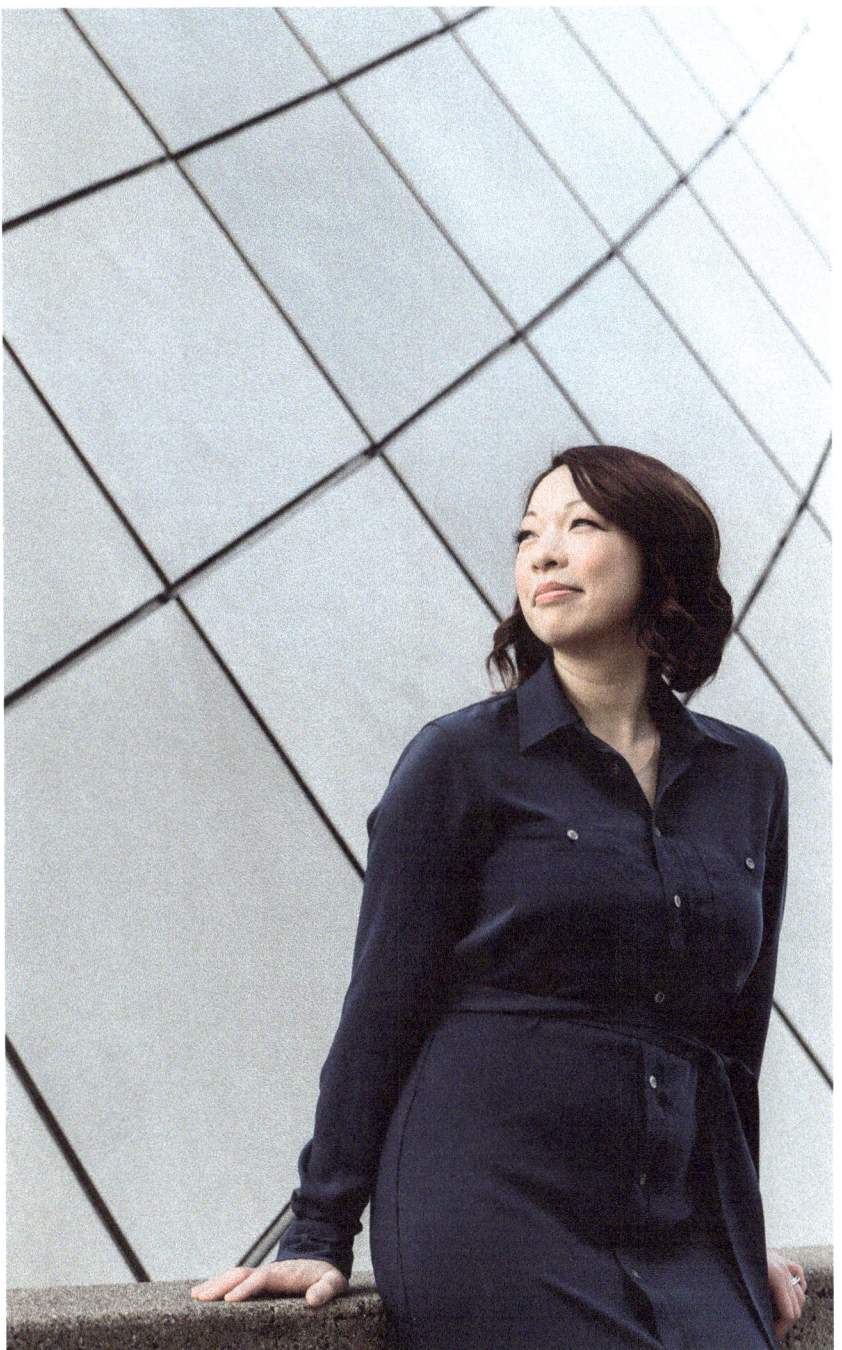

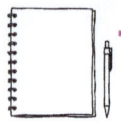

Creating Your
Personal Impact Statement

Creating a personal impact statement is another powerful way to identify the difference we want to make in the world. To create your personal impact statement, fill in these blanks:

> I am a _____(metaphor), who _____ (impact I want to have).

For example, this is my personal impact statement:

- I am a trail guide and trail blazer, who inspires others to be their most joyful, bold, and authentic selves, and who, in turn, inspire others.

And here are some others:

- I am the wise sage, who opens the door of possibility for others.
- I am the woman by the sea, who invites others to join her to dance and sing and lead fulfilled lives of service.

Allow yourself to be fully free and creative as you brainstorm your metaphor, your impact, and then your impact statement in your Workbook.

Once you have drafted your personal impact statement, say it out loud five times. What do you feel? Rate your inspiration level on a scale of one to ten, with one being the lowest, and ten the highest.

Ask yourself these questions:
- What number do I rate my current impact statement?
- How can I alter my impact statement to make it a nine or ten, if it's not already there?

Make these changes, then post your impact statement next to your list of core values. Start each day saying your personal impact statement out loud to yourself. By doing so, you are setting your intention for who you want to be and the impact you want to have that day and in your life. As a badass woman in medicine, knowing exactly who you are, what you stand for, and what you want your impact to be are crucial steps to creating a life you truly love.

Remember: You must start by deeply knowing your value, your worth, your non-negotiables, your priorities, and your Why. Without these important guidelines, you will be drifting without direction. Know that for many of us— particularly for women physicians—these concepts are new and may feel strange. Leadership training is rarely incorporated into medical training even though it is sorely needed. As doctors, we are the leaders of our teams, clinics, and hospital, and yet we receive little to no preparation for this role in our careers. Therefore, we must foster a clear understanding of who we are and what we stand for, so we can lead from the inside out.

Reflection Questions

1. How do you relate to Dr. Shruthi's story at the beginning of the chapter?
2. What are your top five core values?
3. What is your Why? If you're not there yet, what themes emerged as you brainstormed?
4. What is your personal impact statement? What metaphors resonate for you? What impact do you want to have?
5. What have you noticed about yourself as you worked through these exercises?
6. How do you view yourself as a leader in your personal and professional life?

CHAPTER 5

DEVELOPING
SELF-COMPASSION

Dr. Shruthi's Struggle with Self-Criticism

Dr. Shruthi is someone who always comes through for her friends, colleagues, and family. Despite all her successes, though, she is plagued by constant fears to "not screw it up." That any small wrong step could kill a patient. That she would never be able to hold her head up again should a patient die while in her care.

She approaches each day on a mission to always do her very best work and do absolutely everything possible for her patients. She is meticulous in everything she does, from the moment she scrubs in and out of a case, to rounding on patients, to her documentation. She believes this is who she must be to survive and compete with her fellow residents—especially as a woman surgeon. But her expectations are unachievable because she feels her work could always be better. In an effort to achieve perfection, she is wearing herself out.

Two years into her life as a surgical attending, she is exhausted and sees no end to her struggles. She is overly demanding and impatient with everyone: her husband, her colleagues, her staff, but most of all, herself. "How could you be so stupid? What were you thinking? Who do you think you are? Stop being so weak!" These thoughts run through her head on a continuous loop. She double- and triple-checks everything she does out of fear of making a mistake. She has received feedback from staff—especially female staff—that she is "too demanding" and "too abrasive," and she doesn't know whether to scream with anger at the injustice of these comments, or just give up and cry. She gives 200% to her patients all the time, but people around her don't seem to notice or understand how hard she is working. Most of all, she is unable to give herself grace in any way. To Dr. Shruthi, there is no room for error. No room to laugh or be herself. No room to breathe. She feels like she is living in a cage.

The Pressure to Perform

Can you relate to Dr. Shruthi's life? Have you experienced similar thoughts and experiences? I certainly have. While not a surgeon, I still felt the same pressures to perform, to achieve, to always be "on" and to give 200% every single day. And the thoughts that ran through my head thousands of times a day were very similar to Dr. Shruthi's. What an awful way to live! But that was my internal world, too. Now, when I remember those thoughts, they seem like foreign words.

We must remember that our lives are shaped by the thousands and thousands of thoughts we have each day—our ongoing internal monologues. And what we say to ourselves in those thoughts triggers our emotions, our behavior, how we show up in the world, our relationship with others, and, most of all, our relationship with ourselves. What a different kind of life we would have if we chose to be kind to ourselves instead of giving ourselves the constant, negative self-critique that is the reality for so many of us as women physicians. To others, we might be kind, compassionate, and caring, but we must also be mindful of what we say to ourselves.

The Power of Self-Compassion

Kristin Neff, PhD, a ground-breaking researcher in the field of self-compassion, and Christopher Germer, PhD, a pioneer in the integration of mindfulness and psychotherapy, have published a large body of work on self-compassion. Through extensive research, they have shown that having self-compassion is highly correlated with increased resilience and decreased depression and anxiety; significantly improves relationships; and improves quality of life (Neff and Germer, 2012). The core principle of self-compassion is to treat yourself with the same compassion that you would someone else, or, as Brené Brown writes in *Dare to Lead*, "Talk to yourself as you would to someone you love".

How would you speak to someone you love? What kinds of phrases would you say to your good friend, if she had a tough day? How would you want her to feel? My hunch is you would want her to know she is doing great, she is a good person, she is loved, and she is worthy, even if something has not gone well. I think you also would want her to understand she is heard, seen, and appreciated for who she is. That she is loved unconditionally. You probably would say phrases like these:

- "You're doing the best you can. And the best you can do is more than good enough."
- "You are enough as you are."
- "I love you."

How We Speak to Ourselves

Now, take a moment to think about how you talk to yourself, especially when you are stressed at work, at home, or in between. Are your words

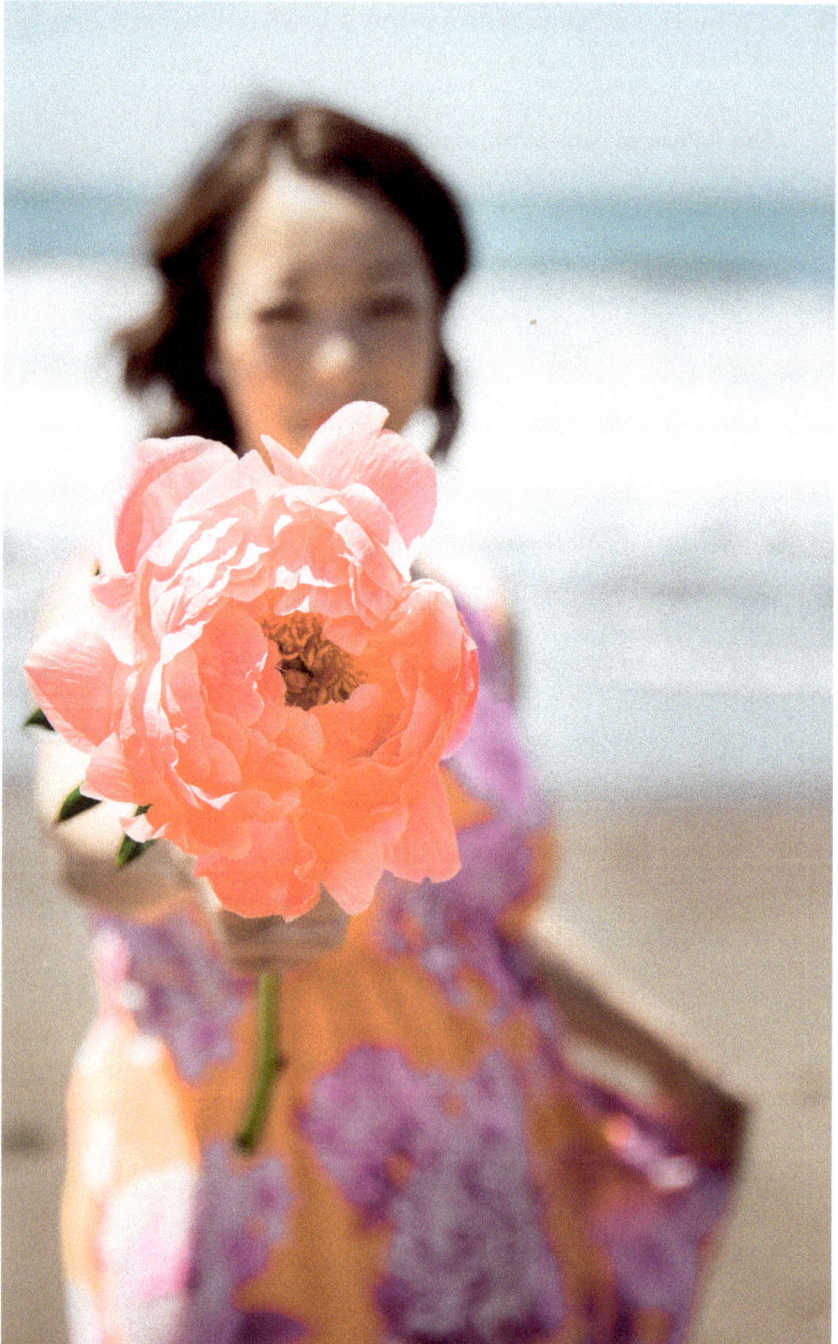

kind, compassionate, and loving, like the words you would say to your good friend? Or are they the words of a harsh critic—angry, impatient, irritated, annoyed, frustrated, and critical?

Take Ten Minutes

In your Boundaries Journal, write down all the things you are saying to yourself in your head right now. Then look at this list of your inner thoughts. Are they predominantly positive or negative thoughts? What tone of voice do you use when speaking to yourself? Is this voice warm and loving or high-pitched and nagging? How would your voice be different if you were speaking to your good friend instead?

Visualizing Compassion

As we have discussed previously, visualization is a powerful tool. It helps us access an inner knowing and creativity that provides us with the right answers.

Let's take a moment to visualize compassion. What does compassion look like for you? What does it feel like? Who is someone in your life who embodies and models compassion? Take a deep, slow breath, and picture this kind, wise person sitting in front of you. What is her presence like? How does she handle conflict, stress, money, work, and her insecurities? What phrases does she say to herself throughout her day? What would she say to you, right now?

Taking the time to slow down and visualize how we want to be is a crucial step toward creating a purposeful life. You can choose how you show up in the world. You can decide to be the compassionate, wise woman you just visualized.

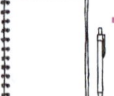

Phrases to Say to Yourself

Below are some phrases to try when you find yourself being hard on yourself. I use them myself and recommend them to my coaching clients:

- "You're doing great, sweetheart."
- "You're doing the best you can."
- "Oh, well!"
- "I love you."

Practice saying each of these phrases out loud. Which of them resonates for you? Brainstorm what other phrases would help you show yourself the compassion and grace you give to others using the worksheet in your Workbook.

The Power to Choose

Earlier, we explored your core values, your Why, and the impact you want your life to have. Now, add this: What kind of thoughts do you want to have toward you? We must take the time to slow down and notice what we say to ourselves, not just because I'm telling you this or because Drs. Neff and Germer told you to, but because deep down you are longing for more freedom, love, and joy in your life. By continuing to be harder on ourselves than anyone else, we are not allowing ourselves to experience all the love, joy, and connection that is possible. We're not treating ourselves with the same compassion that we bestow on our patients, friends, and colleagues. And unless we treat ourselves with that same kindness and grace, we are not showing up fully as the women, doctors, and leaders we are capable of being.

I know you are a kind, compassionate, resilient, and hardworking woman. Realize that you are more than enough, just the way you are. You will be able to set clear boundaries once you realize this truth and fully accept it.

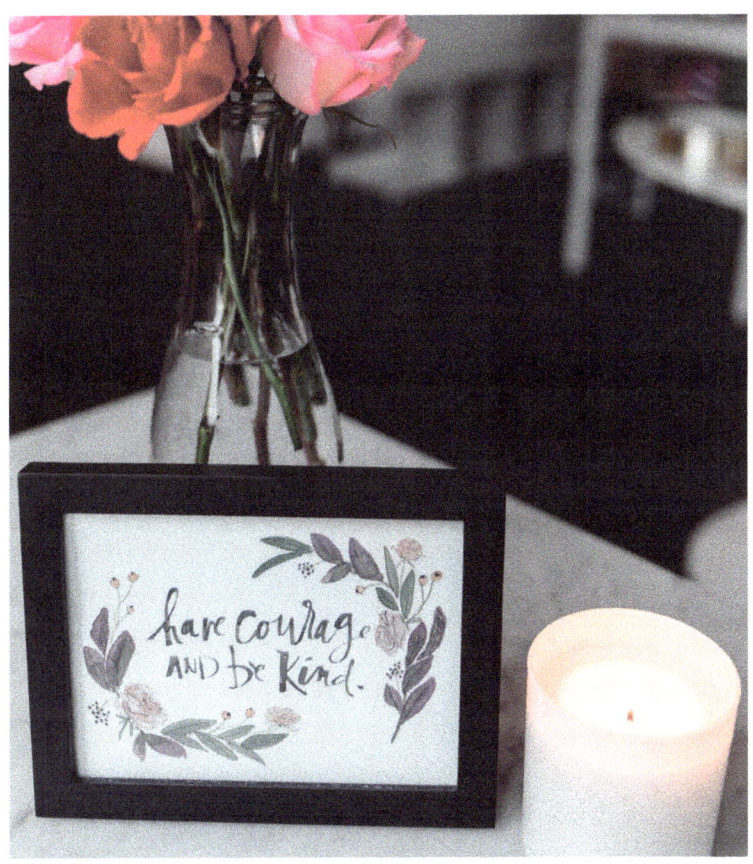

Reflection Questions

1. Let's try another brainstorm exercise. Using your Boundaries Journal, take Ten minutes to write every thought that is in your head at this moment. Do a free write and don't take your pen off the paper. Write it all down. After ten minutes, sit back and examine the quality and tone of the words and phrases you wrote. Are they kind and understanding? Shrill and critical? Judgmental? Loving?

2. When are you particularly hard on yourself? What do you say to yourself at these times?

3. Who is someone in your life who inspires you to be kind, compassionate, and loving? What is it about this person that inspires you?

4. What do you want to commit to saying to yourself, as if you were a good friend and someone you love? Write these phrases down. Print them out and put them next to your core values, your Why, and your personal impact statement.

CHAPTER 6

UNDERSTANDING FEAR
AND PERFECTIONISM

Dr. Shruthi's Greatest Fear

Dr. Shruthi's deepest fear is that others will realize how much she doesn't know. That she covers up her inadequacies and insecurities with her hard work and drive. That she doesn't measure up as a surgeon. When she thinks back on her life, she is not able to remember a time when she didn't feel this way. From her early middle school years through high school, college, medical school, intern year, and residency, she has always had a nasty voice inside her head, telling her, "You're not good enough." She can't help but compare herself to her fellow surgical colleagues and attendings, who always seem to have it together. They seem to be confident in what they are doing, without the self-doubt and negative internal dialogue that nag Dr. Shruthi.

Dr. Shruthi is harder on herself than anyone else, but she is also extremely critical and skeptical of others around her. "Are they doing what they said they would? Did they do it the right way?" Dr. Shruthi finds herself double- and triple-checking not only her work but also the work of others, looking for faults. She demands perfection of herself and expects those around her to strive for it, too.

Dr. Shruthi's fear of failure permeates everything she does, especially when she has an upcoming challenging surgical case. She can't stop thinking and reading about everything that could go wrong. She worries, "What mistake could I make? How could I kill this person?" These fears fill her mind for days before the case. She has difficulty sleeping and worries that if she makes a mistake, she will be vilified forever by her colleagues and staff. She imagines having to present the case at the departmental Morbidity and Mortality (M&M) conference. Touted as a learning and educational opportunity, everyone knows M&M conferences are designed to point an accusatory finger at the responsible surgeon and provide a cautionary message for all other attendees: "Don't mess up, or you will be next." Dr. Shruthi has seen this happen and doesn't want to be the next surgeon burned at the M&M stake.

I understand Dr. Shruthi's fears, as they were my own for so many years. My hunch is that some—or even all—of this resonates for you, too.

Striving For Perfection

Research about fear and perfectionism reveals fear is a natural human instinct that motivates many behaviors (Adolphs, 2013). Humans initially developed this part of our neuro-wiring millions of years ago to help us survive by protecting us from actual real danger, like saber-toothed tigers, lions, bears, and cheetahs. However, perfectionism distorts this instinct by causing us to be afraid of our inadequacies and failure. With perfectionism, our physiologic experience feels the same as if we were confronted with a pack of salivating wolves: our cortisol shoots up and puts us on high alert. But instead of protecting us as fear does, perfectionism causes us to strive for the unattainable and then to berate ourselves because we do not achieve it.

What does perfectionism feel like for you?

My Quest for Perfection

I remember when I first developed my unrelenting work ethic, drive to succeed, and fear of failure—when I became a perfectionist. As the daughter of strict, and loving, immigrant parents, the values of hard work and excellence were part of my earliest memories. I started playing the cello at age four and soon after added the piano. I gave my first solo recital at age five. By the time I was six, I was told I was musically gifted and praised for my talent, which made me want to improve and perform even more. By the time I was ten, I was practicing the piano several hours a day, trying to perfect every note, tone, and quality of sound. In high school, I got up early to practice the piano for several hours before school and then practiced late into the night, after completing all the homework from the competitive private high school I attended.

Playing the piano developed the perfectionistic streak that I also applied to my life as a student. I strove to be the best in my class at my private school and to get as close to a perfect score on the SATs as I could—which I did—so I could attend an Ivy League university. In addition to practicing the piano, I took on a heavy schoolwork load and was involved in many extra-curricular activities. I rarely slept more than four hours a night. While other teenagers were attending parties and hanging out on Friday nights and weekends, I was at home studying and practicing. I was an exceptional student and pianist, but at what cost? I remember often thinking I couldn't possibly keep going at that pace. I was totally stressed out but didn't know any other way to be.

At a young age, I ran on over-drive and continued to do so for the next several decades while I became a physician. Now, when I coach other women physicians, I often hear them describe a similar overwhelming drive to achieve success and avoid failure that is fueled by a relentless drive for perfectionism.

What were your childhood and teenage years like? When do you remember first beginning to fear failure and strive for unattainable perfection?

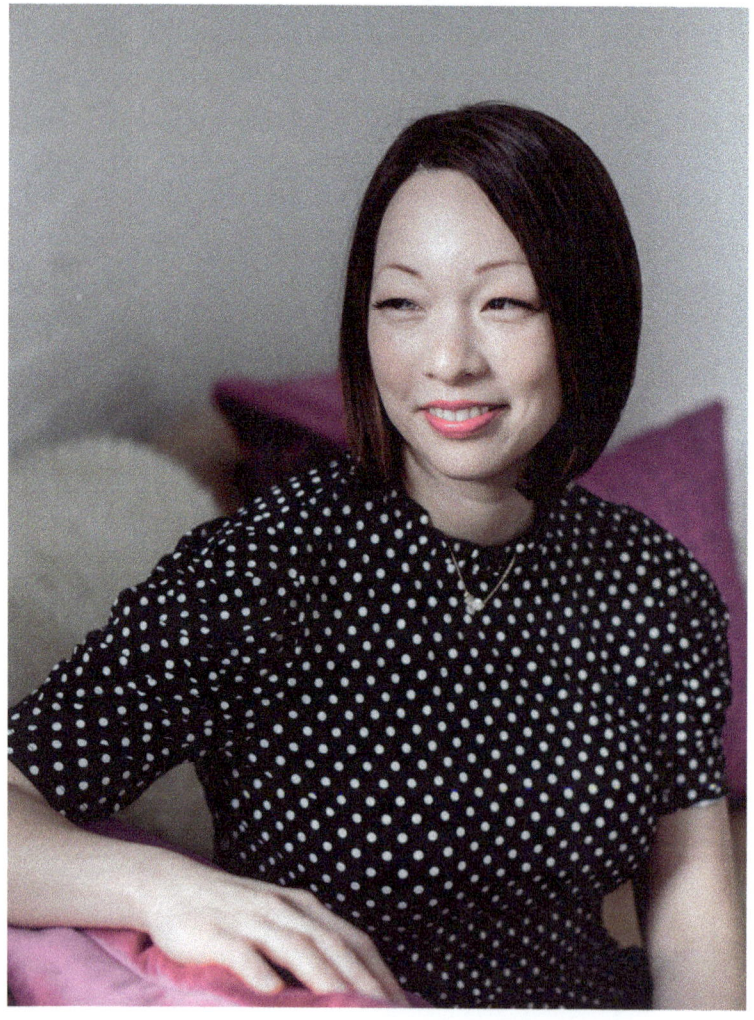

BOUNDARIES *for Women Physicians*

The Plight of Women Physicians

A wealth of data exists about women physicians: How we have improved patient outcomes and have better patient satisfaction scores than male doctors (Tsugawa et al., 2017). How we make less income, spend more time with patients, and spend more time in the electronic medical record per patient than our male counterparts (Melnick, May 2021). How we have higher rates of burnout, higher rates of emotional exhaustion, and a higher risk of suicidal ideation and death by suicide (Dutheil, 2019; Houkes, 2011; West, 2018). How as women physicians, we are innately more nurturing, other-focused, and have higher emotional intelligence (Day, and Caroll,, April 2004). This means we connect more readily and quickly with our patients, and yet we still feel we must work even harder to compete with our male colleagues.

Let's compare one aspect of a doctor's life and look at how it varies for female versus male physicians: the quantity and quality of medical documentation. Research shows that women physicians tend to write significantly more thorough and longer chart notes than men. And then we frequently go back and double-check our work to correct grammar and spelling errors. Our patient histories of present illness are often several paragraphs long, and our assessments before the plan minutely detail our thought processes. As students, we were often praised for our excellent documentation, and then again as interns and residents. This same dedication to over-achievement follows us as we become attending physicians. We continue to strive for perfection with documentation even when it no longer serves us.

Male doctors, on the other hand, tend to write much shorter entries in their charts. This is not to say that they do a poor job recording their patients' histories, assessments, or plans. They just tend to write only what is necessary. How many male physicians do you know who go back and endlessly refine their grammar and notes? Men tend to get the job done with the minimum of effort required and so have more time to devote to other aspects of their medical practice. This sounds like a pretty good idea to me! What do you think? (We will discuss ways to cut down on charting time in a later chapter).

Hiding from Notice

At times, we hide to keep ourselves safe by avoiding notice. A voice inside our head tells us to stay quiet, don't make a fuss, and don't complain, or else others will see us and all of the mistakes we make and thus won't like us. Some call this voice our saboteur, which developed in human beings millions of years ago to protect us from outer danger. We hid in caves to avoid being eaten by saber-toothed tigers. However, what we must recognize is that this saboteur no longer serves that purpose in our modern lives and instead diminishes our potential as human beings, and as women physicians. Our saboteur thinks it's keeping us safe, but instead it is keeping us small and unrecognized.

When do you allow your saboteur to direct your actions? Where in your life do you notice yourself hiding? When do you feel you have to keep quiet for others to like you?

Creating Our Internal Boundaries

Awareness of perfectionism and self-sabotaging fears is the first step toward creating healthy boundaries for yourself. These negative thoughts and emotions don't need to be part of your life. Recognize that these thoughts are completely normal and experienced by every human being on the planet. Then decide if they are serving you by asking yourself these two questions:

- In what ways is my perfectionism hindering rather than helping me?
- What fears are holding me back?

The answers to these two questions are the keys to where you need to focus your energy and create boundaries.

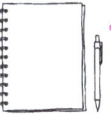

Refer to your Workbook for a list of suggested self-care thought-starters.

Reflection Questions

1. How do perfectionism and fear affect your life?
2. How old were you when you first remember this happening?
3. When you look back on that younger version of you, how do you feel toward her? What wisdom would you impart to her?

CHAPTER 7

DEFINING SELF–CARE
AND SETTING EXPECTATIONS

Dr. Shruthi and Self-Care

Dr. Shruthi doesn't know what self-care means. All she has ever known has been exhaustion: decades of late-night studying in high school, college, and medical school, and then the years of sleep deprivation as she endured 30-hour calls in the hospital. Her education and training have groomed her to put her own needs aside and to relentlessly keep moving forward.

When Dr. Shruthi hears the term "self-care," she feels frustration, anger, and guilt. She thinks self-care is about getting massages and pedicures, going to spas, drinking wine, eating chocolate, reading books, and attending girls' nights out with friends. "How can this possibly be the answer to the severe burnout I am experiencing as a surgeon and physician? I don't have time for self-care. I feel guilty even thinking about it."

Self-Care is Not Just Getting a Pedicure

The very first myth I want to debunk for you is that self-care is all about pedicures and spa dates. Yet self-care is less about getting pampered, and more about saying "no" to the things that do not bring joy or energy. It's about how we protect our most precious resource—our energy—to allow us to be our best, whole selves.

To me, self-care means I must take care of myself and my needs before helping others. Not long ago, I would have felt this was selfish, and I would have felt guilty, but we've all watched the safety video on planes that shows what happens when you, as the responsible adult, do not put on your oxygen mask first: you pass out. And then the young child seated next to you has no one to help her. You can't be of assistance to anyone else if you don't take care of yourself first. The same is true with self-care. You must first satisfy your own needs before you can help others.

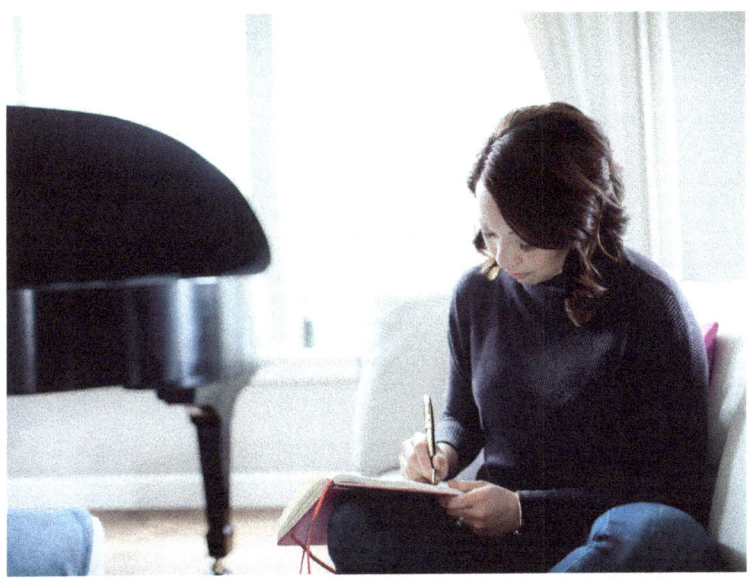

The Basic Necessity of Sleep

Contrary to what we learned in medical school, we physicians need our sleep! A plethora of research reinforces the critical role a physician's sleep plays in patient safety and patient outcomes (Trockel, et al., December 2020). A lack of appropriate sleep is also strongly associated with the increased risk for physician depression, anxiety, and suicidal ideation (Kalmbach, et al., March 2017). Sleep is vitally important, and yet, as trainees, we are forced to go for years without it.

Given the opportunity, the first thing I would change about the medical world today would be a revision of its dangerous attitudes about doctors' sleep needs. I would advocate for physicians to be relieved from taking overnight call, working overnight shifts, or having shifts of longer than ten hours. We all know these changes would require a monumental transformation of our current healthcare system but they would greatly benefit the well-being of doctors and improve the care provided to patients as well. Until then, we physicians must personally take ownership of setting boundaries and making choices that prioritize our sleep.

The Six Pillars of Lifestyle Medicine

According to the American College of Lifestyle Medicine, sleep is one of the six pillars of lifestyle medicine, which also include exercise, healthy diet, stress reduction, connection with others, and avoidance of risky substances. I had never heard of lifestyle medicine, a boarded medical specialty, until two years ago, but once I began to explore this field, which supports long-term health and decreased cardiovascular disease, chronic disease, and mental illness, I had to wake up and pay attention.

The concepts of lifestyle medicine are so simple. And they are exactly the six key concepts we stress for our patients: sleep, exercise, healthy diet, stress reduction, connection with others, and avoidance of risky substances. Yet, I know if we were to poll a room of 100 women doctors most of us would admit to not prioritizing them in our own lives, because our medical training and culture have taught us not to do these exact six things. As physicians, we often are the worst patients. Okay, we are totally the worst patients. The irony is comical.

Defining Self-Care

For me, self-care means I need to sleep between seven and eight hours per night, workout every morning, eat healthy food, avoid alcohol, meditate, play the piano, and spend time outdoors with those closest to me. If I skimp on any of these priorities, I'm not my best self. Instead, I am cranky, bloated, grumpy, and less compassionate. I don't want to be around myself and I don't want others to be around me. Only when I see to my self-care needs do I begin to thrive and become the joyful, loving, woman and leader I want to be. I can create, write, think, reflect, and connect with my deepest and most authentic self. I have so much inside that I want to give and share, but I can't begin to do this with the impact I want to have unless I am taking care of my basic requirements first.

What does self-care mean to you? What changes do you need to make in your life to meet your needs so you will be available to help others? We explored your core values, your Why, and your personal impact statement in previous chapters. Do your self-care priorities align with what you are learning about yourself? How can they be more aligned?

Setting Expectations and Saying "No"

Part of self-care is setting clear expectations with the other people in our lives. The next time you feel the urge to say, "Yes, I can do that," stop and take three deep breaths. Before responding, visualize the wise, kind, and compassionate leader inside of you, and imagine how she would react to the situation at hand. Take all the time you need. If the request for assistance arrives by email or text message, you don't have to respond at that moment. If it comes by phone or in person, tell the other person, "I will think about it and get back to you." While you pause to reflect, ask yourself these questions:

- What do you want to do?
- Do you have to say "yes"?
- Can you say, "No, not right now," instead?
- What would your inner wise leader do?

Keep in mind that when we start saying, "No, I can't right now," instead of, "Yes, I'd be glad to help," it's a big change, and change is almost always uncomfortable. We are not used to saying "no," and other people are not used to hearing us say it either. I know this, as I have experienced it myself. You too will notice that as you begin to set boundaries, the attitudes of the people around you will begin to shift. After you begin to say "no" more often, you'll find that you won't receive as many requests for help. When you take longer to respond to a message or email, the frequency and rapidity of these emails will decrease. And if you keep your door closed at work and are less available, you will be interrupted less often. I'm serious—this works. Try it! And all of this begins with self-care and setting expectations.

Reflection Questions

1. What does self-care look like and mean to you? What needs to be in place so that you can make sure these things happen every day?
2. What expectations do you need to set with others in your life so that you can put your self-care on the top of your to-do list?
3. What kinds of reactions might you receive when you begin to do this? How will you handle these reactions from others?
4. What one action will you commit to today to put self-care on the top of your list? What are you saying "yes" to when you do this? What are you saying "no" to?

CHAPTER 8

CREATING MORE LOVE, JOY, AND FREEDOM. RESPOND, DON'T REACT.

Dr. Shruthi's Transformation

Dr. Shruthi has been following this book's advice and is noticing changes in her life. She has clarified her core values and her Why. With this increased self-awareness, she feels more lightness, too. She recognizes the voice of her inner critic, chastising her for not working hard enough. She gently pushes away those criticisms and the other negative thoughts she has. She notices how her body feels throughout the day and what it needs. She takes more breaks. She realizes when she walks briskly through the hallways, she smiles more. She is receiving feedback from staff that she seems happier and easier to be around these days. "What's been the change?" they ask.

Dr. Shruthi's transformation from a worn-out, short-tempered, and irritable surgeon to a woman who notices herself and the people around her has been gradual. She's not sure when the exact moment of change occurred, but she recognizes that she feels calmer, more centered, and more grounded. She pauses before speaking and then talks slower. She even laughs sometimes. Wow, what a difference from the Dr. Shruthi we first met earlier in the book!

Like Dr. Shruthi's experience, the change to creating more energy, joy, and freedom in our own lives can be a subtle transition over time. As we begin to recognize our core values, our Why, and our self-care needs, this gives us the foundation to create much-needed boundaries in our lives. Without this self-awareness, we are more vulnerable to external stimuli and much more likely to react, rather than respond.

Reacting vs. Responding: Awareness of Our Emotional Triggers

Reacting is the automatic, knee-jerk answer to stimuli whereas responding is a deliberate, thought-out reply. This subtle difference is the key to modifying our behaviors. It occurs in the moments between external stimuli, thought, and emotional response, where we have the greatest power to direct our actions. This space is where we can rise to our highest and best self, achievable by putting our intention in this internal space.

We have much more power over our responses and behaviors than most people realize. When working with women physicians, I've found that using the cognitive-behavioral model of emotion is extremely helpful in illustrating this concept.

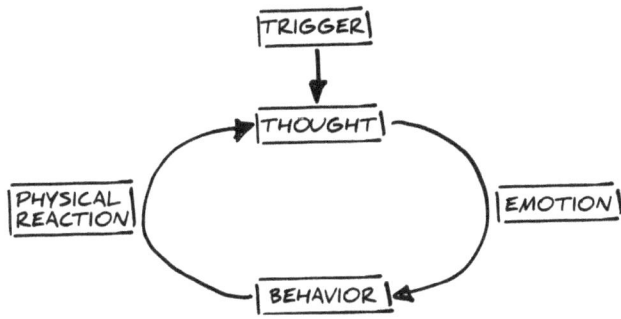

When we are exposed to an external situation or a trigger, we form a thought and then an emotion in quick succession. This happens in less than a split second. Our emotion then drives our behavior, physical reaction, and ultimately the consequence or result of this behavior.

We usually hear about human behavior being modified at the level of the behavior. However, the most effective moment to alter behavior is at the time of the trigger or thought, before we develop a full-blown emotion which then drives our behavior. The space between the trigger and our cognitive reply is where we have the opportunity to respond rather than react.

One of the most common struggles I work on with women physicians is how to regulate emotion. Have you ever noticed how a conflict or situation can trigger a strong emotion within a split second? I help clients recognize what causes them to be triggered with a strong emotion and then what to do about it.

When your nervous system is activated into high gear through an emotional response to a trigger, you are no longer operating from your higher executive functioning state where you can make logical choices to resolve the situation. Instead, you switch to flight or fight mode, reacting in anger, fear, or anxiety, as if confronted by the saber-toothed tiger we met in an earlier chapter. To get yourself out of this triggered state, your need to calm your nervous system. Breathe deeply, walk away from the situation, put down the phone, or leave the room. Do whatever it takes to separate yourself from the emotional stimuli so you can calm down and regain your executive prefrontal cortex functioning. Often it will only take a few seconds or minutes to diffuse whatever you are experiencing. Sometimes—when the situation or stimuli is particularly strong—it may take hours to regain your calm and move on. However, if you find yourself dwelling on a situation for days—or longer—you may need professional help from a coach or even a therapist.

Practicing emotional awareness and regulation is a muscle we must flex every day. As we become more accustomed to noticing our emotions and what we need to bring ourselves to a calmer, more rational, and higher state, we begin to respond to situations rather than react to them because we are more in control. We can show up as our best and most authentic selves, and thus we are modeling self-leadership.

Creating Our Inner Emotional Freedom

We are like an iceberg, with only our actions and behaviors visible to others. Our complex, internal, emotional world lives beneath the surface, hidden from view. We may appear cool, calm, and together on the outside, but inside we may feel completely out of control or trapped.

When we are fully aware of our core values and our Why, we have an anchor to use to live a more congruent and harmonious inner and outer life. We recognize when we feel triggered, upset, down, or angry. Rather than reacting by saying something we will later regret or sending an email that we later wish we hadn't, we stop, slow down, and respond more rationally.

We are human beings, which means we will have strong emotional reactions. We can't beat ourselves up when these are triggered. Just remember we have more control over the space between the external stimuli and the response than you may realize. And when we are living a less reactive and more responsive life, we can set the boundaries we need, which, in turn, will allow us to experience more love, joy, and freedom in our lives and our inner world.

Reflection Questions

1. For the next five days, use your Boundaries Journal to record the details of each time you are triggered with a strong emotional response.

2. When you are in the throes of a strong emotional response, what helps to calm you? Write a list of ten things you can do to calm yourself.

3. Try this 4-7-8 breathing technique, based on pranayama breathing exercises from yoga, a very effective tool to calm our nervous system introduced by Dr. Andrew Weil, a practitioner and teacher of integrative medicine.

   • Set a timer for 2 minutes.
   • Close your eyes and sit comfortably.
   • Breathe in slowly for 4 counts, hold for 7 counts, and then breathe out slowly for 8 counts.
   • Do this for 2 minutes.
   • Notice how you feel before and after this exercise.

4. At this point in the book, what have you learned about yourself? How have you grown?

5. What have you learned that will help you be your best self at work? At home? We will explore these changes further together in the next two sections of this book.

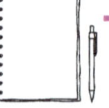

Refer to your Workbook for additional tip sheets.

CHAPTER 9

PROFESSIONAL PATIENT-PHYSICIAN BOUNDARIES

Meet Dr. Angela

Like Dr. Shruthi, whom we read about in the past few chapters, Dr. Angela is a phenomenal doctor. An experienced family medicine physician in her mid-50s, she is deeply devoted to her patients and families. She has cared for several generations of families through every phase of their lives and finds her work tremendously rewarding. She would do anything for any of her patients.

Dr. Angela is known for being so devoted to her patients that she often runs late in the clinic. Then she works into the evening on her charts and continues charting once she gets home. Despite all this, she is often 30 charts behind and has had to work with the administrative leaders of her practice more than once to maintain her privileges because of outstanding billing and charts.

Dr. Angela's patients love her, because they know she will go above

PART III

BOUNDARIES AT WORK

and beyond for them. Dr. Angela gives her cell phone number to her patients and families, so when they don't get what they want from her clinic staff, they can call her directly. It's not uncommon for Dr. Angela to receive phone calls and text messages in the evening and on weekends, and she has helped many patients avoid going to the emergency room after hours. Dr. Angela leaves her pager on 24/7 in case anyone—colleagues or patients—needs to reach her.

Dr. Angela feels like she is doing the right thing by being always available to her patients, but the lack of downtime is beginning to wear on her. She often feels resentful when she receives a late-night phone call from patients. Her staff calls her off-duty and during her vacation time, too, knowing that she will respond, which makes her feel taken advantage of. "Don't they realize that I deserve some time off?" she asks.

Despite her feelings of aggravation, Dr. Angela has never considered ignoring calls or clearly stating to staff and patients that she is unavailable on the evenings, weekends, and vacation time. She feels guilty saying "no" to staff and patients. After all, isn't she supposed to give 100% of herself, all the time? Isn't that what doctors do? Instead of voicing her frustrations, she remains silently resentful.

Can you relate to Dr. Angela's predicament? How much of her life do you see in your own?

Boundaries and Patients

When we think about professional patient-physician boundaries, we first remember what we learned in medical school and our training. We recall all the basics: It is unethical to receive additional payment or benefits from patients. We are not to enter into a romantic relationship with a patient. We must respect patient confidentiality and abide by the rules of the Health Insurance Portability and Accountability Act (HIPAA). We should not become friends with patients or patient family members on social media.

These boundaries protect the patient, but where are the ones that protect us, the physicians?

As physicians, we are taught to be available 24/7. That we are responsible for our patients first and above all else. That we must always go above and beyond and give 100% of our energy in service to our patients—all the time.

To this, I encourage you to just say, "No!"

Because none of this protects us or our ability to take care of ourselves. No law says we must live, sleep, and die for our patients. When considering the age-old dictum, "Do no harm," we need to apply it to ourselves—the physicians—too. I challenge you to honor your needs FIRST. Because unless you take care of yourself, you will not be available to help anyone else.

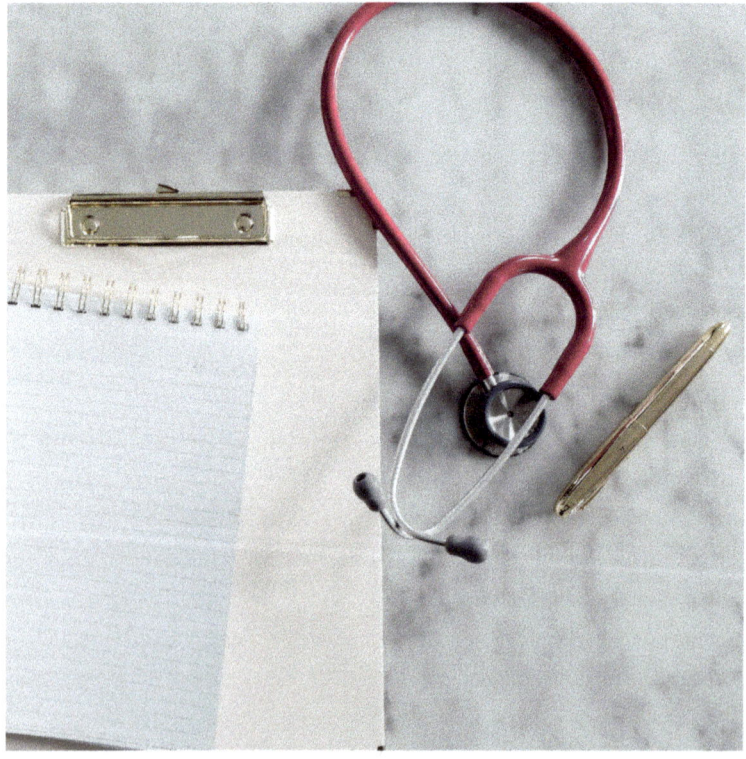

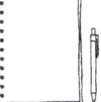

Patient-Physician Boundaries to Consider

Here are some patient-physician rules to consider adopting that are designed to establish boundaries to protect you, the physician:

1. When a patient sends you a long question via your in-basket or a telehealth message, respond that to fully address his needs he will need to see you in person or schedule a telehealth visit. Your response should not be more than one short 50-word paragraph, because you are not paid to be his physician by email or electronic message.

2. While in a clinic, if a patient comes in for one problem and then asks for help with five more, ask her which two problems are the most pressing and then tell her she will need to schedule a separate visit to fully address the other concerns. If you go way over the scheduled appointment time to address all of that patient's concerns, she will assume you will always do this no matter how much time you have allotted for her visit.

3. Furthermore, failing to set time limits with patients will make you run further and further behind schedule, causing patients with subsequent appointments to become upset as they are forced to wait for you. And these delays will have a cumulative effect, too: Your last patient will be livid for having to wait so long. You will finish seeing him after 6 p.m. and will have completed none of your chart notes. Your staff will be angry about having to stay so late. And you will be exhausted, hungry, and spent.

4. Don't provide assistance to your patients that allows them to circumvent going through your clinic. Instead, have them follow the prescribed steps in place for your practice, such as your phone tree, clinic procedures, or hospital processes. After all, if you show them an easier way to get what they need, they will always come to you first. People do this not because they want to make your life difficult, but because they want to make their own lives easier. I call this the **Law of Boundaries Landslide**!

5. Regardless of whether you work in an inpatient clinic, operating room, emergency room, or urgent care setting, apply the same rules: Set expectations and limits with patients from the outset. Let them know you are only available when you are at work or on call. Make it clear no emergency requires you to be disturbed while on vacation. If you set the expectation that you are not accessible and do not respond if you are contacted outside of working hours, patients will learn to respect your boundaries.

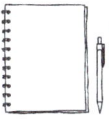

Setting Your Own Rules

What other situations in your patient care work do you find frustrating or draining? Take 20 minutes with the provided worksheet in your Workbook to brainstorm all of these problematic conditions. Now review this list and identify what other boundaries you need to set between you and your patients.

Reflection Questions

1. Which of the physician/patient boundary ideas I've shared in this chapter will help you into your workday?
2. What other boundaries will you set with your patients?
3. What are you doing now that makes physician/patient boundary-setting difficult?
4. What one boundary-setting action will you commit to, starting today?

CHAPTER 10

THE LOGISTICS AND REALITY OF A PHYSICIAN'S WORK LIFE

Dr. Angela's Struggle

As we've seen, Dr. Angela has little separation between work and home: She responds to pages on weekends, regardless of whether she is on call. She even answered text messages and pages when she was on maternity leave!

Dr. Angela used to relish feeling needed. One of the reasons she wanted to become a doctor was that she enjoyed being of service to others. It allowed her to value herself. She has been a helper and a giver ever since she was a young girl.

But now, she is becoming increasingly resentful of all of the extra demands of her patients, staff, and colleagues. She feels she can't possibly do it all and often feels suffocated by the needs of all of these people. She notices her blood pressure rises when she receives a work-related text message on the weekend. Her pager's buzz has become an emotional trigger for her, sending her instantly into anger mode. Once she threw the pager against the wall and broke it. Maybe you've done this, too. I know I have…!

When Dr. Angela is home, she feels she can't relax because of the constant cloud of outstanding charts that follows her everywhere she goes. Even on vacation, she regularly spends time each day writing in them, barely finishing in time to go back to work. Due to this, she feels she is never off work and is irritable and short with her family and friends. Sometimes she hates her life.

Does this sound familiar to you? I can certainly relate, as this was me not too long ago.

No, ladies, no.

Say it with me: "No!"

We must set boundaries between our work and our lives outside of work or the two become hopelessly intermingled to the detriment of ourselves, our co-workers, and our patients. While I am a proponent of the term "work-life integration" rather than "work-life balance"—as we all know there is no such thing as balance—integration is only possible when we set healthy expectations and boundaries. With these boundaries, conflicts between work and the rest of your life are avoided, and the rest of your life is no longer consumed by work.

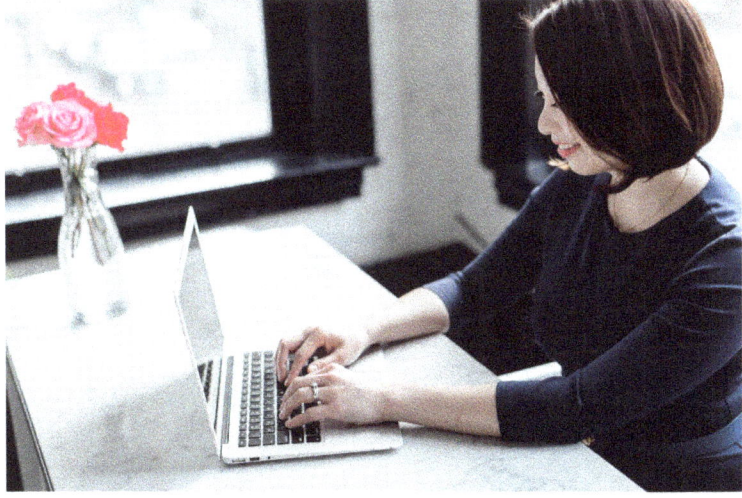

Work Boundaries to Consider

Here are some rules for you to consider implementing as you work to create the boundaries necessary for a healthy integration of your life at work, home, and everywhere in between:

1. Turn off your pager whenever you are not working. This means if you are an outpatient provider, turn off your pager from 5 p.m. to 8 a.m. on weekends and while on vacation. If you work shifts or non-traditional daytime hours, make sure your pager is off whenever you are not at the hospital or on call.

2. Put your phone on "do not disturb" on your days off. People who need you for a true emergency can still reach you (by calling you twice and by-passing your phone's do not disturb setting!). Everyone else can wait.

3. Don't open your Electronic Medical Records (EMR) when you are not at work unless you are on call. EVER. (More on this in the next chapter.)

4. Don't give out your cell phone number to staff or colleagues. If you do, expect them to call or text whenever they need you. Remember: they do not know your work or vacation schedule.

5. If you must give out your cell phone number, then be prepared if someone contacts you off hours:
   - Say, "I'm not working or on call, please refer to the on-call schedule and contact that physician."
   - Or say, "I'm on vacation and not available."
   - Or don't respond to the text or call. If it is a true emergency, the caller will find the right person to help him.

If I Can Do It, You Can Too

I know not responding to a text or call from staff or a colleague will bring on feelings of guilt for many of you. I used to feel guilty, too. It has taken years for me to finally retrain myself and my emotional triggers to not respond when I'm off hours. If I can do it, you can too.

Remember that when you first put these boundaries in place, the change will feel uncomfortable for you and those around you. You are learning to treat yourself the way you want to be treated, and you are training others to treat you appropriately, too. But once you establish these boundaries and stick to them, you will find, after time, people will stop texting or calling you off-hours since they know you will not respond. Instead, they will contact the correct person. This indicates you have successfully trained yourself and them.

Reflection Questions

1. What boundaries do you need to establish to keep yourself from being available all the time to your staff and colleagues?
2. What needs to change so that when you are off-hours you are truly away from work?
3. What one action do you commit to today to establish and maintain these boundaries?

CHAPTER 11

ELECTRONIC MEDICAL RECORDS (EMR) AND CHARTING

Dr. Angela and the EMR

During medical school and residency, Dr. Angela was known for the completeness of her notes. She prided herself on documenting every part of the patient's history and every treatment detail so anyone opening the chart would know the full story. She felt she should—and did—provide this service to her patients. She often received feedback from colleagues that her notes were the most comprehensive they had ever read, which gave her a sense of achievement and made her feel proud.

Now that she's in practice, Dr. Angela increasingly feels her notes have taken over her life. Her charting is never done. She is always behind on responding to her overwhelming mountain of in-basket messages, results, telephone messages, notes from staff, and prescription refills. She is frustrated because too much of her time is spent in front of the computer instead of with her patients. She often thinks, "Why do I have to do all this documentation? It is such poor use of my time. This has nothing to do with taking care of my patients."

Dr. Angela works on charts on weekends and often declines social engagements to finish her notes. She feels resentful about her EMR, remembers the days of paper charts, and laments how much easier it was to finish charts back in those days.

Too Much Documentation

Does Dr. Angela's story sound familiar to you?

I sure can relate as this was my life, too, until I realized that I could change things; I could drastically reduce the number of hours I spent charting and doing EMR by debunking some of the myths we'd been taught in medical school.

The first myth I would like to dispel for you is that your worth as a physician is tied to the thoroughness of your notes. It isn't. There is absolutely no reason for you to spend hours and hours perfecting your notes so they read like a Dickens novel.

As third- and fourth-year medical students, we were drilled on how to write a good patient history and physical. As interns and residents, we were chastised when our notes were not written in full sentences, when key pieces of the history of present illness were left out, when our assessment did not include a thorough and well-thought-out differential diagnosis, and when our treatment plan did not include a full plan by systems. When we entered the real world, we brought our good student habits with us—to our detriment. We continue to write notes fit for a novel, which are unnecessary and a waste of our time because once we are done with our training, it doesn't matter how well-written our notes are. Overly detailed notes benefit no one and take up way too much of our valuable time.

C=MD/DO

As women physicians, we have been groomed to write beautifully thorough notes—to do A+ work all the time. Ladies, let me tell you this right now: your C-level note-writing work is more than adequate to record the information necessary. You passed your courses in medical school, graduated, and have earned the right to place "MD" or "DO" after your name. So, you no longer have to write Shakespearian-grade patient notes. C-level work will do because C= MD/DO!

The next time you find yourself writing a chart note that takes you longer than ten minutes, realize you are writing too much. I am serious. All your notes need to do are: (1) get the key points of the patient visit across, (2) provide enough detail to protect you legally, and (3) provide whatever documentation is required to bill at the appropriate level. That's it. What makes you an excellent physician is the quality of the patient care you provide, not whether you have beautifully crafted full sentences in your notes, so permit yourself to do less than perfect documentation. You no longer are being graded on your chart-writing abilities.

When I finally absorbed this nugget of information after 20-plus years in medicine, I was able to conquer my struggle with charting. Because I was once more than 300 charts behind. Yes, I am completely serious! But by implementing the simple mindset shift to C = MD/DO, I am now able to finish all of my notes each day and leave work before 5 p.m.

If I can do it, you can, too.

Change Is Uncomfortable

I know C=MD/DO is a difficult concept for women physicians to accept because it means we have to change. And, as we've discussed previously, anytime we force ourselves to change and form new habits, we become uncomfortable. But just because we are uncomfortable

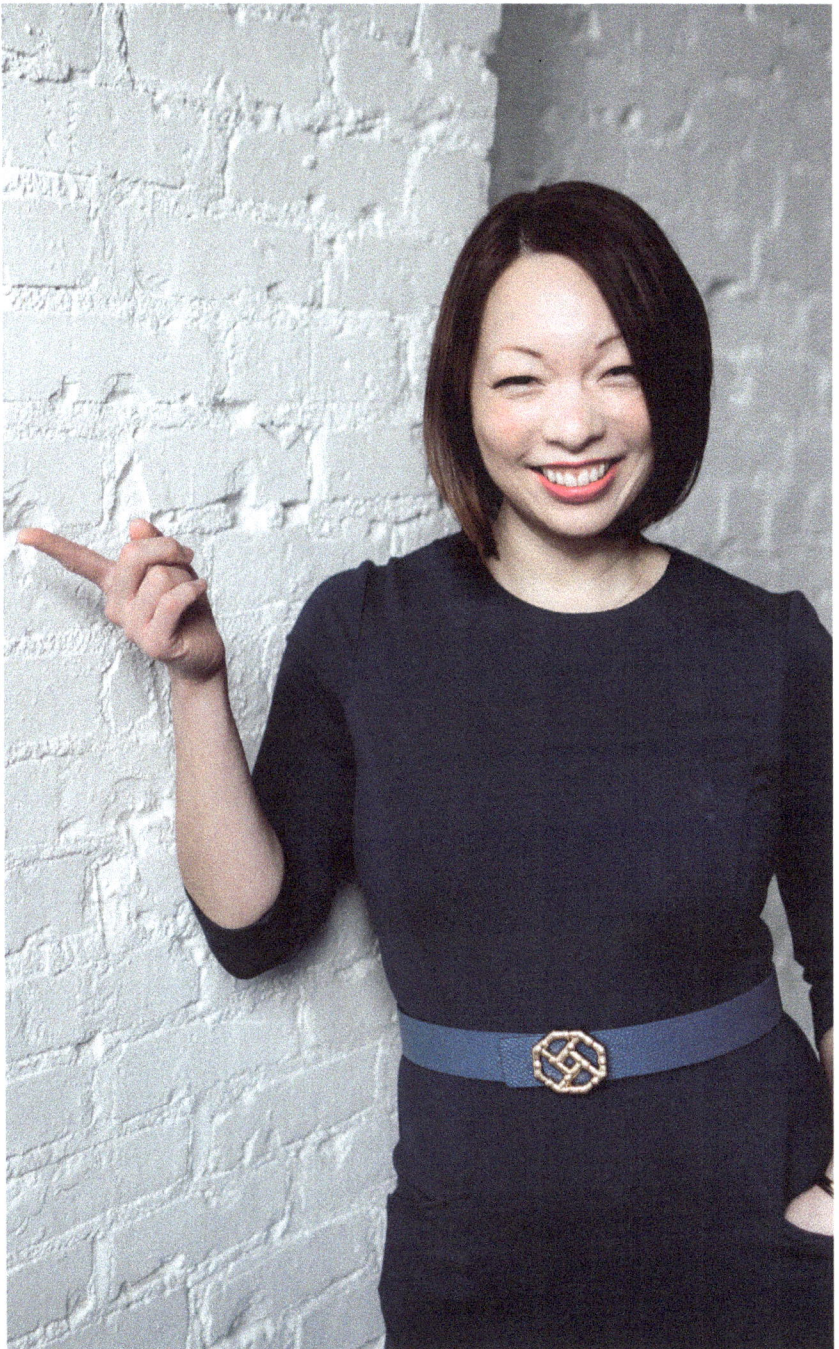

doesn't mean we should avoid change. If we want to set boundaries and live a life of freedom, we must do the uncomfortable work of changing old, unproductive habits.

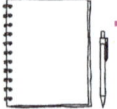

EMR and Messaging Boundaries to Consider

Here are some rules to consider adopting to create EMR, charting, and messaging boundaries for yourself:

1. If you are working in an outpatient clinic, finish the notes immediately after you see the patient. There are two reasons for this: (1) this is when the information is freshest in your mind and thus will take you the least time to document, and (2) this forces you to be concise and spend as little time as possible—less than ten minutes per note—otherwise you will be late to see your next patient.

2. If you work in an inpatient, emergency room or urgent care setting, the same rules apply! Finish your notes immediately after you see the patient. Do it when the patient encounter is fresh. This is what I do when I'm rounding on the inpatient service. And I help my multidisciplinary team to do the same, so that they complete their documentation and orders after each patient too. At the end of rounds, we are all done with our notes and task lists! A win-win all around!

3. When you notice yourself slipping into "good girl student mode," repeat this phrase: C = MD/DO. Post it on your computer monitor to remind yourself that

C-level EMR work is all that you need to do to be a successful, practicing physician.

4. Let me clarify: I'm not advocating doing crappy work. But I am challenging you to allow yourself to do average work when only average work is needed (that is, for charting and your EMR). So, rather than over-stressing yourself to do A+ work all the time, you can choose for yourself when it is appropriate (such as when you are interacting with patients, caring for a family, explaining a difficult diagnosis, or delivering tough news).

5. If you have charts left to finish at the end of the day or shift—as we all do on occasion—give yourself a deadline. Make it a game. Set your timer for 30 minutes and challenge yourself to complete all of the charts in that amount of time. My hunch is if you only allow yourself 30 minutes, you will get them done in 30 minutes. If you allow yourself three hours, it will take you three hours. Remember Parkinson's Law, which states that work will expand to fill the time allotted.

6. If you are in an outpatient setting, if there is something urgent that needs your immediate attention, ask your staff to call you or let you know in person rather than sending you an in-basket or email message.

7. Otherwise, designate specific times for checking your in-basket messages and emails and let your staff know in advance that you will be checking messages during these times only. Perhaps go into the office 20 to 30 minutes early each morning, to clear out any of these messages before your day starts. Then

DO NOT open the message tab again until your next scheduled in-basket and email time, maybe from 12:00 to 12:30 p.m. Then at the end of the day, from around 4:30 to 5:00 p.m., take care of as many messages and emails as you can. If you are not done at 5:00 p.m., leave it. Yes, leave it. Anything in an in-basket or email message can wait 12 hours until you return to work the next morning.

8. Designate 20 to 30 minutes during your lunch or mid-shift break to actually take a break. Leave your office, even if all your charting and other work is not done. Go outside if the weather is good. If not, take a walk through the building and visit a friend or colleague on another floor. The 20 minutes of movement will give you the energy to push through the rest of your shift and help you be more on task.

9. If you don't finish all of your charts, billing, and messaging during the workday, DO NOT take them home with you. Instead, come in 30 to 45 minutes before your next shift or early the next morning and crank them out before your day begins. You will be infinitely more productive, efficient, and focused when you do this versus trying to write notes at night after the kids go to sleep, which is much-needed wind-down time for you.

10. If you will be out of town, on the inpatient service, or slow to respond to messages for some other reason, post an out-of-office message on your EMR and your email. This will let others know that you are not available and that you will respond when you are

back in the office—and ONLY when you are back in the office, not from home at night or on the weekends.

If you do all of the above consistently, I guarantee that you will not be writing notes or responding to a backlog of email messages on your next vacation.

Reflection Questions

1. Which of the suggested rules for setting EMR and messaging boundaries appeal to you the most?
2. Which feel the least comfortable to you? Notice this, it may indicate what boundaries you need to work on most.
3. What do you commit to doing so that you can live a life free of the burden of your EMR and emails?

CHAPTER 12

COLLEAGUES AND STAFF

Dr. Angela and Other People

While Dr. Angela struggles with making herself unavailable to her patients when she's off-hours, what she has even more trouble handling is how to separate herself from the needs of her staff and colleagues. Since she always seems eager to help and take on projects, her co-workers rely on her to do many things above and beyond her regular scope of duties. She's become the go-to person everyone in the office relies on.

Since Dr. Angela is known to be easy to talk to and a good listener, staff come to her with their problems. It's not uncommon for her to have a co-worker visiting her office to ask for advice over lunch or at the end of the day. Often these conversations go on for 40 or 50 minutes, consuming Dr. Angela's lunch hour or the time she could have finished her charting. To avoid this, sometimes she keeps her door closed, but staff members just open the door when she does not answer it. Dr. Angela used to think this was a good thing—that her staff felt very comfortable with her—but nowadays she feels frustrated and annoyed about her lack of private time.

Her clinic is experiencing a staff shortage, and two of her physician colleagues are out on maternity leave. Because of this, her remaining colleagues are stressed and come to Dr. Angela to vent their frustrations. She feels bad for them, so she volunteers to take extra weekend calls to reduce their loads. "After all, isn't this what a good person and colleague does?" she thinks. But then she regrets saying, "Yes" and feels weighed down by the needs of everyone else at the clinic, who always seem to want something from her.

Can you relate to Dr. Angela's situation? How are your experiences with your co-workers and staff similar or different from hers?

Who's on the Lawn Outside Your Metaphorical House?

At the beginning of this book, we discussed the metaphor of the house as representing you, the fence as your boundaries, and the lawn as the buffer between you and the outside world. When I described my house metaphor, I mentioned that I felt like I had patients, staff, colleagues, and everyone else sitting in camp chairs on my lawn, waiting for me. I was afraid to look out of my windows for fear of them noticing me and asking me for something. I knew I would have a difficult time saying, "No."

In your house metaphor, are there people camped out on your lawn, waiting for you to pay attention to them and help them with their needs? Are some of them your staff and colleagues? How do you feel about them being there? What would you like to change about your relationships with colleagues and staff?

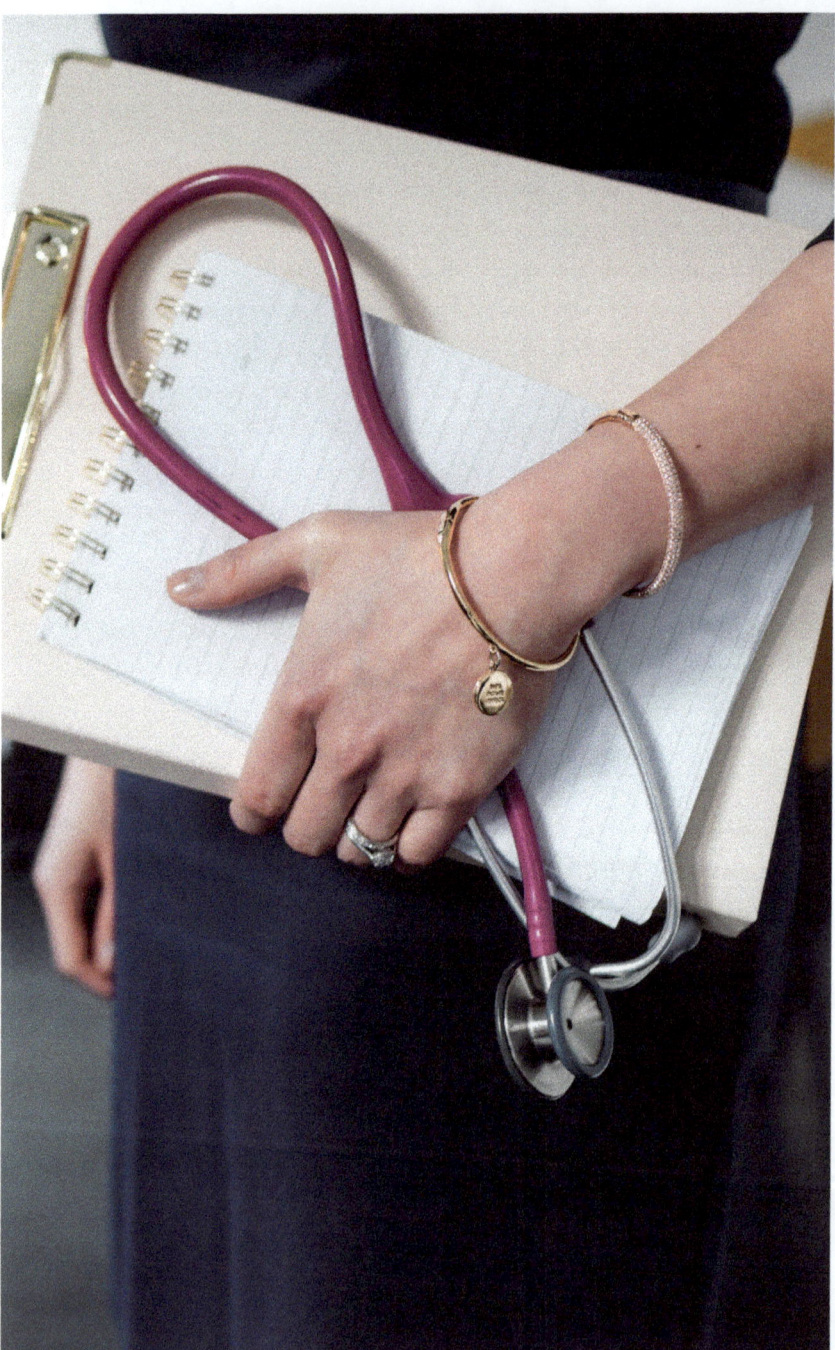

Work Boundaries to Consider

Here are some rules for you to consider using to create boundaries with your staff and colleagues:

1. Remember that your value is not measured by how helpful, giving, or available you are. Your value is you, and you are enough without having to please anyone around you.

2. When you say, "no" to your colleagues and staff, you are setting a boundary that shows them how you want to be treated—which is valuable information for them, and models good, healthy boundaries that may help them to set their own boundaries.

3. If you have a problem with co-workers walking into your office without knocking first, lock your door. This will train them to not enter your office without your permission.

4. If a staff member or colleague comes to you unannounced, looking to get advice, vent their frustrations, or lament about their woes, gently but firmly tell them you have work that needs to be completed and are not free to talk at that time. Don't offer to talk with them later—that may encourage them to repeat their behavior. Just say, "I'm not available now."

5. Do not apologize to your co-worker for being unavailable to counsel him. After all, you are protecting yourself—your most important resource— and others should respect you for this. You are also modeling good boundaries to your co-worker, who likely needs help setting boundaries, too.

6. When you receive a request to help cover, do extra shifts, or do more call, don't respond. Yes, I'm

serious—don't respond. If your staff and colleagues aren't getting what they ask from you, they will solicit someone else. Eventually, they will stop asking you = The Law of the Boundaries Landslide.

7. If you're worried that enforcing some of these boundaries will make you seem unfriendly, cold, or impersonal, I get it. I've been there, too. Let your colleagues know in advance that you are trying to make changes in your life so that you can be more present at work and in your life outside of work. To maintain good relationships with your staff members, chat with them for a few minutes first thing in the morning or at the beginning of your shift, letting them know that you are trying to focus during the workday or shift on completing your work so that you can leave at a reasonable time. Then return to your office, close your door, and get to work. If you work in a shared office or an open charting space, you can consider wearing headphones (not ear buds) to signal to others when you are not available. At the end of the day or shift, when you are done with your work, again spend a few minutes speaking with your co-workers and staff.

8. Another reason to go on a walk break during lunchtime or your mid-shift break is that if you are out of sight, you won't be asked to solve your co-workers' problems or answer additional questions.

I promise if you implement some of these strategies, you will see a difference in your day-to-day work experience in no time.

How can you incorporate some of these boundaries in your work environment, regardless of your work setting?

Reflection Questions

1. What boundaries do you need to create with your staff and colleagues so the yard of your house metaphor is clear of people clamoring for your help?
2. How will creating these boundaries with people at work help you feel less emotionally triggered?
3. What action will you commit to today that will help you set boundaries with your co-workers?

CHAPTER 13

PUTTING IT ALL TOGETHER
AT WORK

Dr. Angela is Catching On

After adopting the rules and boundaries suggested in this part of the book, Dr. Angela no longer dreads going to work. Now she gets her charts done most days. In the morning, she goes into work 45 minutes early to complete any remaining work and clear her in-basket. She no longer opens her EMR or email messages at home at night, even when her work is not completed. She has more energy throughout her day, especially when she goes on a walk at lunchtime. She feels less annoyed by staff and colleagues, maybe because they are bothering her less.

Without the burden of dozens of uncompleted charts, Dr. Angela feels lighter during her workday. She still slips back into old habits by writing too much detail in her chart notes, but then reminds herself that C=MD/DO. Her C-level work is more than good enough to be a practicing physician.

Dr. Angela now keeps her office door locked so she doesn't need to worry about unwelcomed visitors. The clinic staff seems to be catching on, too, and no longer rely on her for counseling services. Occasionally, she passes staff whispering in the hallway and worries, "Maybe they are talking about me." But then she realizes she is not there to serve the staff's needs. She and the staff are there together to care for the patients. This is a freeing thought.

Now her colleagues email and text her much less often. When she receives an unreasonable request for coverage, she doesn't get annoyed; she simply doesn't respond, and then they ask someone else. Because her colleagues no longer come by at the end of the day to complain and vent to her, Dr. Angela feels much less frustrated with them. Working each day feels much easier, lighter, and contains less drama.

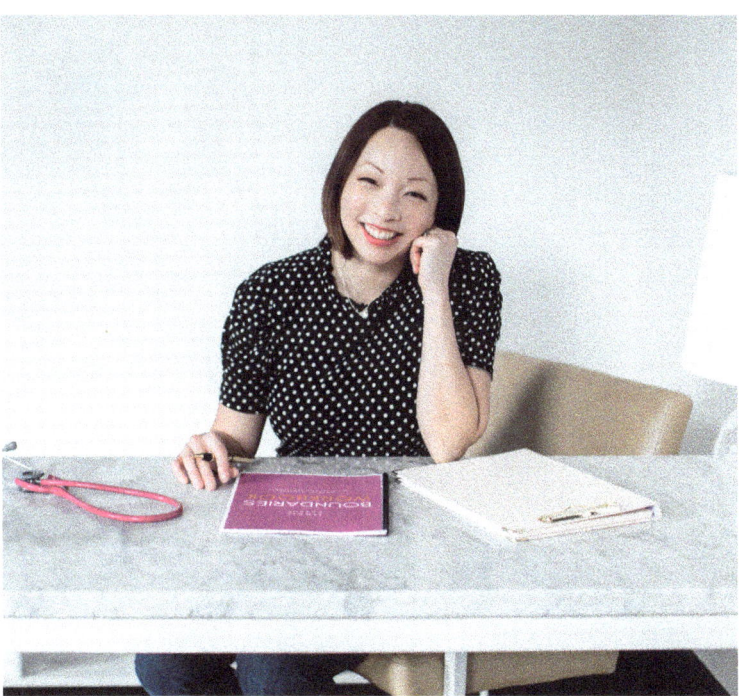

This is What I Want for You

Freedom, healthy boundaries, and ease at work—this is what I want for you, because I want you to not only survive but also thrive as a female physician. I want you to rise above the universal stressors that women doctors face in the healthcare workplace, so you can care for patients the way you long to care for them, lead your teams and departments the way you long to lead them, and live a life that you love—all made possible by intentionally set the right boundaries at work.

I want you to love your life, because you are an incredibly well-trained, hard-working physician who has dedicated the last several decades of your life to this noble profession. I want you to love your career, because our world needs you and the gifts you have to offer as a doctor and as a human being. I don't want you to become one of the 40% of women physicians who quit or are forced to go part-time within six years of finishing their training (Paturel, 2019). Instead, I want you to make healthy choices for your life from a fully resourced place of strength, not from a place of struggle. Setting the boundaries we've discussed so far is essential to help you no longer be a victim to the healthcare system we work in and, instead, will allow you to make the system work for you.

Reflection Questions

1. What is your biggest take-home point from this part of the book?
2. What can you do today to begin to create boundaries to protect yourself during your workday, whether you work in a clinic, hospital, emergency room, urgent care, intensive care unit, or operating room?
3. I want you to have the power to no longer be a victim of our healthcare systems, but instead to make our systems work for you. How does that statement resonate for you?

**WATCH VIDEO MESSAGE
FROM TAMMIE**

PART IV

BOUNDARIES AT HOME

CHAPTER 14

MULTIPLE ROLES

Meet Dr. Amara

Dr. Amara doesn't know how to handle her life. She and her husband, Ron, are the parents of three young children. Ron works part-time from home as an information technology consultant and is the primary caregiver for the children, while Dr. Amara works more than full-time as an internal medicine hospitalist and the internal medicine program director of a large university hospital.

Dr. Amara loves mentoring the residents and teaching at the university, which is why she accepted the position in the first place, but she doesn't love having to constantly put out fires by responding to daily issues with the residents, program, and faculty. She's also responsible for disciplinary meetings with residents and interns, and she serves as the mediator in disputes between faculty and residents. Even while she is on-service as a hospitalist—where she works eight shifts a month, seeing upwards of 20 patients per day—she receives texts, emails, and calls about residency problems. Dr. Amara is finding it increasingly difficult to stay afloat with all that is required of her at the hospital and the university, not to mention the load of responsibilities she has waiting for her at home.

When Ron and she decided to have children, he agreed to take on the bulk of the family and household responsibilities during the day while Dr. Amara said she'd handle the nighttime duties. To do her part, Dr. Amara pushes herself to leave work by 5 p.m. every evening. Sitting in traffic during her 50-minute commute home, she responds to the phone calls and text messages she missed throughout the day—not a relaxing drive. The moment she walks in the door, all three children cling to her. She then cooks dinner for everyone, serves it, cleans up the kitchen, bathes the kids, reads to them, and tucks them into bed. While Ron stretches out on the couch watching Netflix, Dr. Amara takes a shower, pours herself a glass of wine, and sits down at her desk to answer her email, write grants, finish notes, and complete anything else she hasn't gotten to during the day at work. By 11:30 p.m. she begins to nod off and heads to bed, joining Ron who has already been asleep for an hour. When her alarm goes off at 5:00 a.m. the next day, she gets up and repeats the same exhausting routine all over again.

Dr. Amara is cranky and tired all the time. She feels like everyone is constantly demanding something of her, and she never has a moment to herself. For the past ten years, she's tried—and failed—to lose the extra 40 pounds she added to her small frame having three babies. She feels disgusting, fat, tired, and old. "This must be what happens when we turn 40," she says to herself. Dr. Amara hates her life but doesn't know how to make it better. She feels like she has no idea who she is anymore.

How do you relate to Dr. Amara's story?

Fulfilling Multiple Roles

Like Dr. Amara, all of us women physicians fulfill multiple roles in our lives. We are physicians, leaders, and mentors at work, and then perhaps mothers, wives, and/or partners at home. Like Dr. Amara, we have been brought up to think that we should have full, demanding careers during the day, and then come home to cook dinner, clean the house, and take care of our families at night. I believe we can have it all—careers and family—but this doesn't mean that we must do it all on our own...and run ourselves into the ground in the process.

If you are fortunate enough to have a good partner in your life, regardless of whether he, she, or they works full-time, part-time, or not at all, one of the most important lessons to learn is how the two of you can share the load at home. If you don't have a supportive partner or are a single parent, you can ask for help from extended family members or friends. Or, you can hire help. You may feel guilty asking or paying for help because you think it's your responsibility to take care of your family and your home. That's what a mother/wife/woman is supposed to do, right? But for you to fulfill your life as a doctor, you must share your home load.

One of the first rules of boundaries we must understand if we are to take control of our own lives and careers as women physicians is that there is no 'supposed to' or 'should' in this life. This contradicts what we've been taught because, as women, we have been brought up to believe that we are supposed to take care of everything and that we should be a helper at all times. There is nothing wrong with helping others, as long as you do not allow yourself to become a servant to everyone's needs except your own. As we discussed in earlier chapters, you must recognize and satisfy your own needs before you address the needs of others.

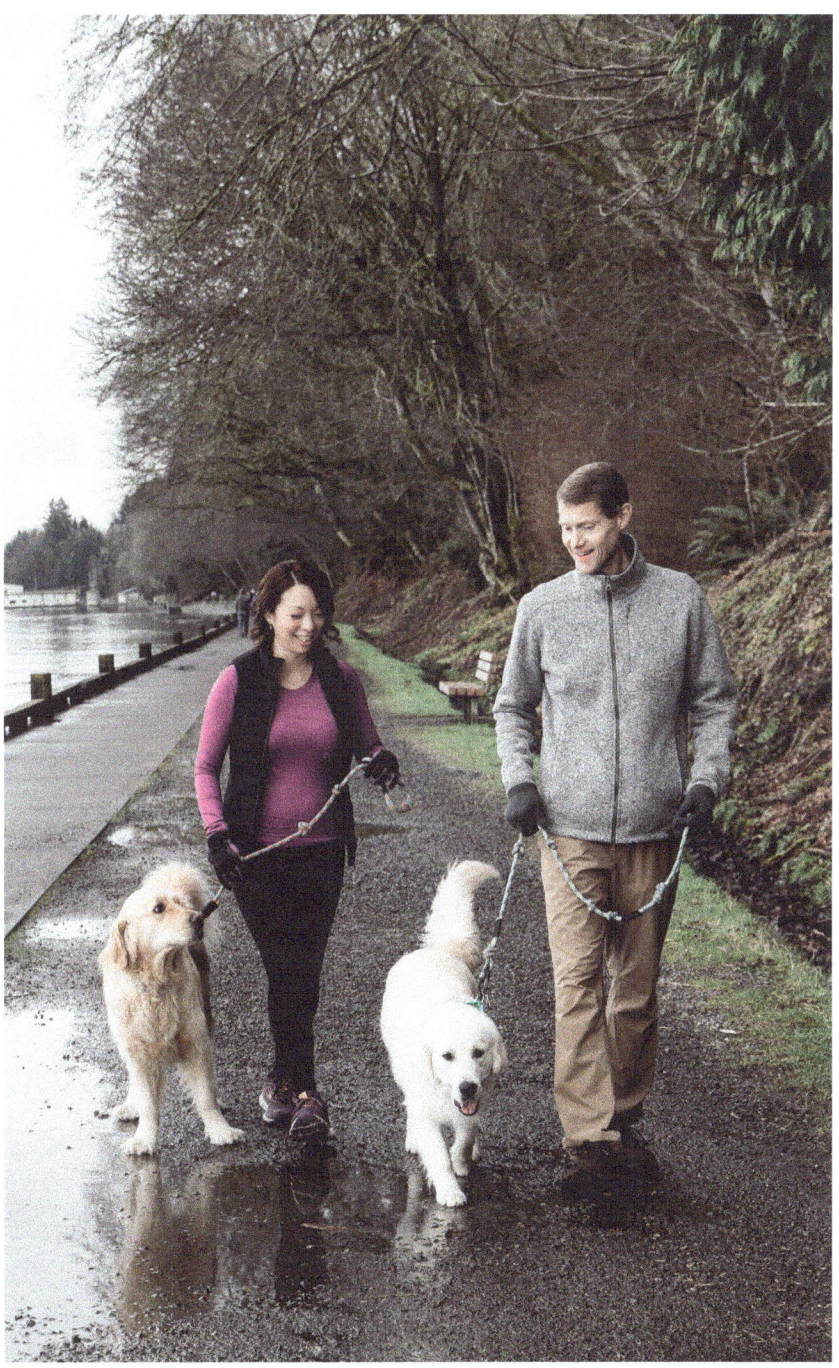

Home Boundaries to Consider

As you create boundaries in your home life, consider adopting these rules:

1. Just before you leave work, turn on your "out of office" messages on your EMR and email services. Then, as you walk out of the door, set your phone and email notifications to "do not disturb" so you are unavailable the moment you leave the building. Your drive or commute home is sacred, alone time for you.

2. On your drive home, do something relaxing that allows you to decompress. Listen to your favorite podcast, an audiobook, Spotify playlist, or Headspace meditation. Do whatever you will enjoy as you commute.

3. Before you enter your home, do something that makes you feel centered and helps you transition to your role at home. Go for a brisk walk, meditate, or listen to calming music. Even two minutes of 4-7-8 breathing that we learned in Chapter 8 can make a huge difference. Adopt this as your end-of-the-workday ritual every single day.

4. Once you get home, be at home. Unless you are on call, don't respond to any more work emails, text messages, EMR, or pager calls. They can wait until you return to work the next day.

5. If you have a partner or a spouse, share the load at home with him or her. Remember: There is no supposed to or should when it comes to your responsibilities as a working woman physician.

So, when you come home already exhausted from your workday, divide the dinnertime and evening responsibilities equitably.

6. Don't be shy about enlisting the help of grandparents or other family members, too. When asked, they probably will enjoy assisting you.

7. Start a dinner-sharing program in your neighborhood where families take turns cooking meals. If seven families sign up, you will only need to cook once a week.

8. Utilize carpools. Take turns with other parents to provide your children rides to sports events, dances, and orchestra practices. This gives you and the other parents much-needed breaks from the constant grind of pediatric taxi service.

9. Whenever you can, hire help such as a house cleaner, yard worker, or nanny. Schedule a grocery delivery service. Hire a virtual personal assistant. Get a babysitter every week so you and your partner can go out or you can have some time to yourself. By doing these things, you are not only off-loading some stressors from your life but also providing valuable and meaningful work for people who need it. Like most doctors, you probably have a mountain of debt including student loans, a mortgage, car loan, and credit card bills and are averse to spending more money to hire help. But consider the alternative: doing everything yourself and exhausting yourself in the process.

10. Once you've made it to wind-down time at the end of your busy day, actually allow yourself to wind

down. This can be gentle stretching, an evening yoga or exercise class, meditation, watching TV, reading a book, taking a bath, or doing whatever you find relaxing, calming, and centering. If you take the time to wind down rather than work late into the night, you will be remarkably more refreshed, energized, and productive the next day.

11. Go to bed at a reasonable hour. Aim for 7 to 8 hours of sleep per night. Remember: Sleep is much more important than we were led to believe while in med school!

You got this, friend. I know you can do it!

Reflection Questions

1. Of the at-home rules we discussed here, which will you try?
2. What other boundaries do you need to create for your life at home?
3. Think back to your core values and your personal mission statement. What boundaries will help you to align with these core parts of who you are?
4. What steps for setting these boundaries do you commit to doing today? How will you hold yourself accountable?

CHAPTER 15

HOUSEHOLD RESPONSIBILITIES

Dr. Amara's Struggle with Household Responsibilities

Dr. Amara has begun to implement some of the at-home boundaries mentioned in the previous chapter but worries she is dumping too much responsibility on Ron, her husband. After all, when she gets home, he often tells her how tired he is and how much he needs a break. She doesn't know what to do about all of the household chores like cleaning, laundry, and paying the bills. Up until now, they have mostly been her jobs to take care of.

When Dr. Amara arrives at home, she often finds their house in a state of chaos with piles of dirty laundry, books, toys, and sometimes trash covering the floor. Dr. Amara can't stand the mess, so as soon as she walks in the door after work, she cleans in a frenzy and continues to work non-stop until she collapses into bed, with no time left over for self-care or relaxation. Her weekends are spent doing laundry, scrubbing toilets, and trying—usually unsuccessfully—to catch up on all of the other household chores that were neglected during the week. She feels overwhelmed by them all of the time.

Overseeing family finances, paying bills, and managing the children's appointments are other tasks that generally fall to Dr. Amara, too. Sometimes Ron helps, but when she double-checks his work, she often finds errors and so has to redo whatever he has done. For example, when he makes appointments for the kids, he often forgets which of their activities fall on what days of the week and so will schedule a dentist appointment at the same time as soccer practice. When Dr. Amara calls the dentist to reschedule, she is frustrated because she could have taken care of the matter much faster on her own.

Dr. Amara feels overwhelmed by her life. By the end of the night, after the kids are in bed, she is done. She has no energy left even to speak with Ron.

Can you relate to parts of Dr. Amara's story?

Overwhelmed By Household Responsibilities

Finding a solution to Dr. Amara's problem is difficult. The burden of the household responsibilities experienced by today's modern professional working women is well-documented. While 57% of American women have paying jobs (US Bureau of Labor Statistics, 2021) and 75% of these working women are employed full time (US Bureau of Labor Statistics, 2017), they are still eight times more likely than men to be primarily responsible for household duties and childcare (Germano, *Forbes*, 2019).

Within the medical profession, women now comprise 51% of students in medical schools (AAMC, 2019), yet we are only 35% of practicing physicians. Four out of ten women doctors either switch to part-time or quit medicine altogether within six years of completing our residency training (AAMC, 2019). The reasons for this are complex, but one cause is the societal expectations we still grapple with which pressure us to shoulder the lion's share of the household duties in addition to all of our responsibilities at work.

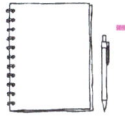

Household Responsibilities Boundaries to Consider

Here are some ideas to use to create much-needed household responsibility boundaries in your life:

1. If you are a woman physician and a single parent, you must take care of yourself so you can care for your children and so you all may thrive. Think about who can help you with your household responsibilities: a daycare center, family members, neighbors, a nanny, or a babysitter. Don't forget about self-care: you need your own life with some days and nights off just for you. So, it's not only okay to ask for help, it's necessary.

2. If you are in a relationship, be honest and open with your partner about the various tasks that need to be done. If you are a dual-physician household, discuss the realities of your pressures at work and how you can equitably share home responsibilities. If you have a non-physician partner, make sure to speak and listen to each other about what you both need and expect, regardless of gender or occupation.

3. Clearly define the responsibilities of you and your partner at home and then resist the urge to double-

check each other's work. Chances are, it will be good enough. If your partner consistently does a poor job, hire someone to help. There is no need for you to do it all on your own.

4. If you have children, remember they are watching you to learn how to treat others. With your partner, model the relationship you want your children to have with their partners someday. If you have boys, show them that men are responsible for taking care of the house and the family, too; that both parents are equally responsible for the load at home. If you are a single parent, model what it looks like to ask for and receive help from others, and that all the responsibility does not fall on you just because you are a mother.

5. And if you do have children, don't forget to assign some of the household chores to them, too. Having them do chores will lighten your load and provide them with valuable lessons in responsibility.

What other boundaries could help you get your home life in order so that you can be the best, unfrazzled version of yourself every day?

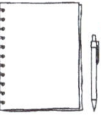

The Power of the 4 Ds

In *The Power of Focus* (Vintage/Ebury, 2001), Author Jack Canfield describes the 4 Ds of time management and prioritization: Do, Defer (Delay), Delegate, and Delete (Drop). When I coach women physicians using this framework, they place way too many tasks in the "Do" category, so I've found this version of the 4 Ds to be much more helpful: Drop, Delegate, Delay, and Do Less. Using this second version of the 4 Ds, complete this:

1. In the provided worksheet in your Workbook, write all the household responsibilities that stress you out, overwhelm you, or drive you crazy.
2. Apply my version of the 4 Ds to all of the items on your list. Yes, all of them. Next to every single item write either Drop, Delegate, Delay, or Do Less Of.
3. Notice which tasks emerge as your highest priorities and evaluate whether they are in alignment with your core values.

Reflection Questions

1. What boundaries will you adopt to help you deal with your household duties?
2. If you are in a relationship, what will you discuss with your partner concerning domestic responsibilities?
3. Who will you ask to help you with these tasks?
4. In what way does the 4 Ds exercise alter your opinion of your household responsibilities?
5. What changes will you make today that will help you resolve these issues?

CHAPTER 16

FAMILY AND FRIENDS

Dr. Amara is Responsible for Everyone

Not only is Dr. Amara busy juggling all her responsibilities at work and home, but also, she is the go-to person for support for extended family and friends. Neighbors frequently drop by for a meal or to say hello in the evenings and on weekends. But even when she's feeling tired and doesn't want to deal with other people's problems, she never says she is busy and can't help them right now, as she always feels like she is being judged and doesn't want to worsen their opinions of her. One neighbor remarked, "Ron is such a good husband. You're so lucky he is happy to stay home and help with the kids. What a great father! Don't you feel bad missing out on the kids' activities so much? It must be so hard for you." Comments like this hurt, because Dr. Amara does feel guilty about being a full-time working mother and not always being available for her children and husband.

Recently, Dr. Amara's aging father, Larry, has suffered from some medical issues. Her mother often calls and texts Dr. Amara—the only doctor in the family—for instructions on how to care for him. Dr. Amara's two younger sisters also call her for advice, relying on her as the wise, responsible, eldest daughter. They constantly seek counsel about some drama related to their work, husbands, or parents. Their brother, Ryan, the baby of the family, has trouble holding down a regular job and frequently reaches out to Dr. Amara for money, and so is an additional source of stress for her.

Dr. Amara's children also require extra attention. Her oldest son is in second grade and struggles with behavioral issues at school. He has been diagnosed with ADHD. Her three-year-old son has frequent temper tantrums in daycare. Both schools often call Dr. Amara at work when issues arise during the day, even though Ron is more available since he is at home with their one-year-old daughter.

Dr. Amara feels like she can't catch a break.

Can you relate to Dr. Amara's life? What boundaries do you think she needs to put in place to help her deal with the unreasonable expectations of her friends and family members?

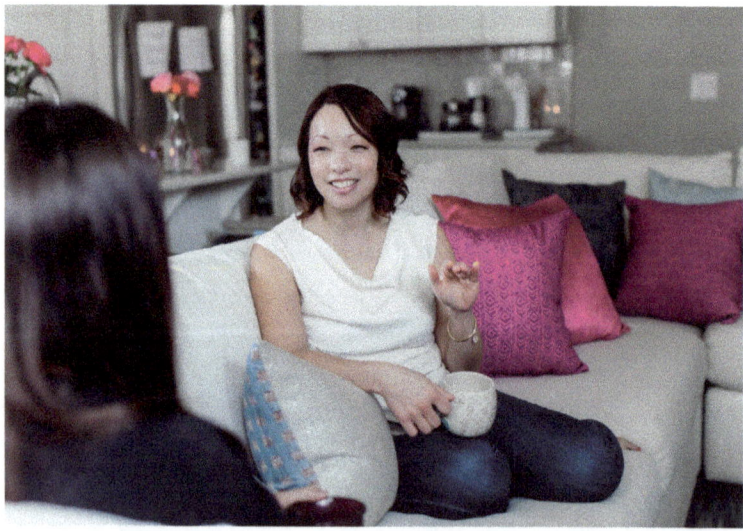

Other Difficulties Women Physicians Face with the People in Our Lives

Women physicians encounter many difficulties when they try to set boundaries with people in their personal lives. Nearly every woman doctor I work with feels she must be everyone's caretaker, helper, and supporter. When a neighbor needs help, the physician drops everything and rushes to support him. When a childhood friend calls because she is struggling with a failing marriage, the doctor is there for her. When the director of her church community asks her to bake twelve dozen cookies for their upcoming church picnic, she feels guilty for not being able to attend the event—she has extended office hours that day—and so makes all of those cookies. When her kid's soccer teammates need a last-minute ride to the game, she goes out of her way to get them all there.

As physicians, we are so used to being helpers, givers, and providers of advice. After all, our medical occupations require us to cultivate those very traits. Because of this, family, friends, and neighbors feel safe with us and often will lean on us to solve their troubles. Sometimes I feel I wear a sign that says, "Ask me to help you with all of your problems!"

Do you feel that way, too?

Boundaries to Consider
with Family and Friends

Here are some rules for you to consider using to set clear boundaries with family, friends, and children:

1. Let go of the guilt. You simply cannot be there for everyone at home and outside of work, so stop feeling guilty about it, set some limits, and be happier right now. By being a thriving woman physician, you'll become a better partner, mother, neighbor, daughter, and friend.

2. Realize you don't have to be everything to everyone, and you have the right to say "no." In fact, by setting your boundaries, you are doing your friends and family a service. You are modeling what healthy boundaries look like and are showing them how to treat others with dignity and respect.

3. If you have a stay-at-home partner or one who works part-time and so is more available than you during the daytime, ensure that your partner is listed as the primary contact for any issues related to your children. If their schools continue to call you first, either don't pick up or remind them calmly and kindly to call your partner instead. If both you and your partner have demanding work schedules, take turns being the primary contact or delegate the responsibility to a different family member or nanny. You don't have to be the sole responsible party all the time. In fact, by delegating, you are giving others in your life the opportunity to be of service to someone—a gratifying experience.

4. Realize that you don't have to be available to help friends and extended family members all of the time. And recognize the fact that this applies even when you feel guilty about not being available.

5. Gently but firmly let folks know when you are and are not available. And then uphold these boundaries. If you don't, be assured others will continue to encroach on your personal time and space.

6. With aging parents, share the responsibility of caring for them with siblings. You don't have to be the one to field all of the calls and text messages just because you are the doctor in the family. And other siblings will appreciate the opportunity to help your parents, too.

What other boundaries do you need to set with the other people in your life?

Reflection Questions

1. Who is draining your energy? Which of the above suggestions would help you curb that?

2. Who brings you joy and energy? How can you spend more time with these individuals?

3. What boundary-building steps will you commit to today that will help you in your relationships with extended family and friends?

CHAPTER 17

BOUNDARIES AROUND MONEY

Dr. Amara and Money

Dr. Amara was raised to be generous and giving. So, when her younger brother, Ryan, asks for financial help, Dr. Amara usually sends him money. She also assists her aging parents with their expenses due to their limited income. She even bought them a car last year when their old Volvo finally broke down. When the whole family gets together for vacations or reunions, Dr. Amara often pays for others' hotel rooms or meals. After all, she is the eldest daughter and the doctor in the family, so they all think she can afford it.

Dr. Amara's generosity doesn't end with her extended family. She loans money to college friends who are unemployed or need cash for an emergency even though they never pay her back. Of course, Dr. Amara always says, "Don't worry about it," because she thinks that's what she's supposed to do, but she finds herself burning with resentment when these same friends reach out to her again and again for more money. "What am I?" she wonders. "A bank … or maybe a charity?"

Dr. Amara is drowning in financial worries. She is the main breadwinner for her family, so it's up to her to pay their mortgage and other major household expenses. But she still has $250,000 in medical school debt that she is paying off more slowly than she'd like. And she worries about saving for her three children's college tuition, and her retirement. She is so exhausted all the time and wants to work less but knows she can't afford it with their family's current financial responsibilities.

Financial Stressors and Physicians Today

Financial matters are a key stressor for physicians today. By the time we graduate from medical school, we incur an average of $250,000 to $300,000 in student loan debt (Educationdata.org, 2021). And as trainees making only slightly more than minimum wage, many of us accumulate considerable consumer credit card debt, too (AAMC, 2021; Medscape, 2020). No wonder we later feel trapped by our jobs; we must work long hours if only to pay back our loans.

After our training, many physicians work in disadvantaged areas for the National Health Service or non-profit organizations to qualify for public service loan forgiveness, but this requires years of commitment at low-paying jobs. We dream of the day when we'll be able to finally live a comfortable life as a doctor, and no longer live paycheck to paycheck. Throughout our training, we were forced to delay our gratification, not being able to afford a decent car, apartment, or other nice things. So, once we become attendings, many of us fall into the trap of living beyond our means.

It's no wonder we feel stressed by financial concerns. As doctors, we are perceived as being rich, but if you add up your assets and then subtract your student loans, mortgage, consumer debt, and financial obligations to family and friends, you probably are nowhere near as well-off as people think.

The next time you feel pressured by guilt to give someone money or donate to an organization, stop and reflect. Do you have the means to give away money right now? Or are you only causing harm to yourself by delaying paying off your student debt and mortgage, and not saving for your children's college tuition? What about your retirement? Are you putting away enough money so that you will be able to retire at a reasonable age and phase in your life? Do you want to have to work until you're 80 years old because you can't afford to retire? My hunch is no.

Financial Boundaries to Consider

Here are some ideas to consider when creating boundaries concerning your money:

1. Please remember that you are not a bank or a charity. Unless you are already financially independent (meaning that, you could retire tomorrow), be judicious with your giving.

2. Set reasonable financial limits and expectations with family and friends. Relationships—especially with family members—are complex and messy enough already, so try to avoid adding money to this mix.

3. When your giving is motivated by guilt, take this as a sign that you are acting on a sense of obligation— a should—and realize that your gut is telling you to say, "No."

Reflection Questions

1. In your Boundaries Journal, write a list of all the areas in your life where money comes into play. Does one, some, or all of these areas cause you discomfort or stress? Circle them.

2. Which of these items are you doing out of a sense of obligation? Mark them with a "G" for "Guilt."

3. To reduce the stress associated with your finances, consider the financial items marked with a "G." Which one is your first priority? What boundaries will you set to alleviate this issue? How about the other guilt-inspired items on your list?

4. Visualize yourself two years from now, with all of the "G" items gone from your life. How do you feel? How has your life changed?

CHAPTER 18

PHYSICAL AND EMOTIONAL SPACE AT HOME

Dr. Amara Feels Bombarded at Home

Dr. Amara rarely enjoys alone time at home. Even when she takes a shower, she has company. Her kids barge in to talk to her. Their golden retriever, Sally, pokes her nose through the shower curtain to bring Dr. Amara a toy. Even Ron, her husband, frequently leans his head in to ask her questions. Dr. Amara seldom has a moment to herself, which causes her to feel bombarded.

How do you relate to Dr. Amara's lack of personal space? Do you feel a lack of privacy due to the others you live with? When was the last time you had alone time to think and breathe?

Feeling Bombarded By Others

Whether we are introverts, extroverts, or somewhere in between, we all need quiet time to ourselves. I am a self-professed extrovert who gets a lot of energy from being with others, and yet I love my alone time. When I create space for myself and allow my body and mind to rest, I feel recharged and my creativity blossoms.

Earlier in the book, we worked together to create a physical and emotional safe haven for you at work. You need your own space at home, too.

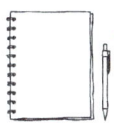

Physical and Emotional Space Boundaries to Consider

Here are some ideas for you to consider when implementing much needed physical and emotional boundaries at home:

1. Have clear rules for your family members. If you are being bombarded by family members while taking a shower, cooking, or trying to work in the office, set some limits. Let them know that you are not to be disturbed at certain times or when you are in a specific space. We all deserve to have some time and space for ourselves.
2. Perhaps your boundaries can look something like this:
   a. Whenever you retreat to your bedroom and the door is closed, the kids can't knock unless it is an actual emergency.
   b. If you are in the bathtub de-stressing in the evening, everyone must leave you alone.
   c. If you are preparing food in the kitchen and don't want the kids' help, they must remain out of the room.

3. Designate a You Space. This could be a separate room, a space in the basement, part of the attic, or a spot outside on your porch. You can even build a She Shed in the backyard. Regardless of where it is, find a space at home where you can be by yourself and others can't physically see you.

4. Make this You Space comfy and inviting by adding things that make you happy. For me, I converted our upstairs den into my She Cave, complete with live plants, lots of pink and fuchsia pillows, cozy candles, my favorite tunes playing on my mini jam box, and inspiring paintings on the wall.

What other physical and emotional space boundaries do you need at home to feel happy and complete?

Reflection Questions

1. Brainstorm ideas in your Boundaries Journal for your own You Space or She Cave. Where will it be? What will you add to this space to make you feel happy?

2. What rules and expectations will you set with family members—even pets—so that this is a sacred haven for you?

3. What one action will you commit to today to begin to make your You Space a reality?

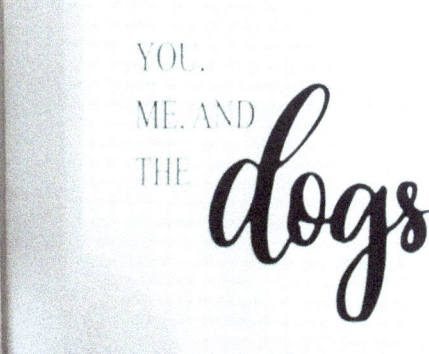

CHAPTER 19

PUTTING IT ALL TOGETHER AT HOME

Dr. Amara's Transformation

After adopting the at-home boundaries suggested in this part of the book, Dr. Amara feels calmer. She allows herself to fully disconnect as she transitions to home during her evening commute. And things are better at home, too. After speaking with Ron about household duties, he is stepping up and taking on a bigger share of the load. They have hired a delivery service that brings all of their family's meals for the week, so neither she nor Ron have to cook. And they've hired a house cleaner so they don't ever have to scrub another toilet.

Dr. Amara has also seen a change in her children, which she considers the most remarkable change of all. As she reduces her stress and becomes more present and connected at home, her children are acting out less and doing better in school. They all enjoy their meal together each evening, and then, as a family, they load the dishwasher and clean up the kitchen together. Once the kids are asleep, Dr. Amara and Ron unwind with each other on their back porch and reflect on the day. They've committed to spending this time together before watching TV. Most often they no longer are interested in watching TV at all. Dr. Amara and Ron now hire a babysitter for a weekly dinner out, and they love this time away together. They are happier and more connected than they have been in years.

Since Dr. Amara now delegates responsibilities to her siblings and no longer lends money to extended family or friends, she feels more content and less resentful about these issues, too. She recognizes that she and her siblings have limited time left with their parents and so focuses on connecting and enjoying her time with them. Because of all of these changes, Dr. Amara is experiencing more freedom to live her life the way she wants to live it ... at last.

Can you relate to this transformation in Dr. Amara's life? What do you think has made the biggest difference?

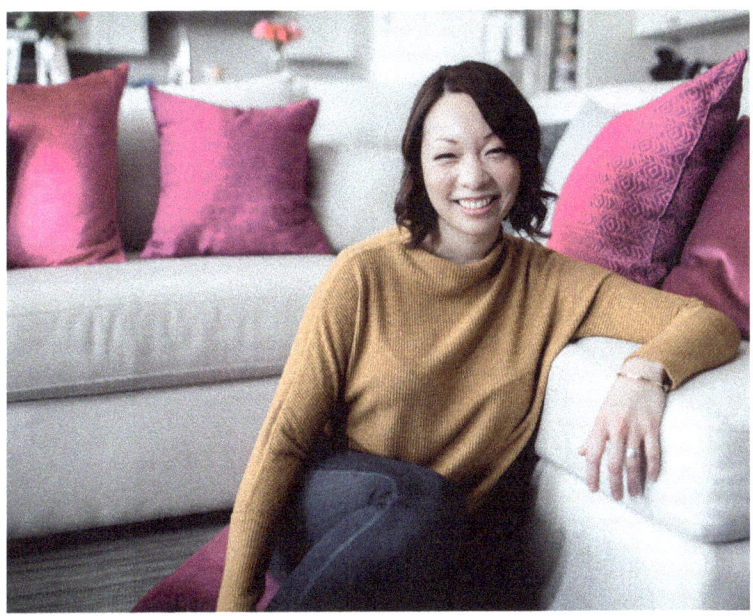

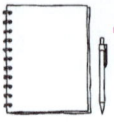

How Establishing Boundaries
at Home Gives You More Freedom

I want you to be the author of your own life by creating
healthy boundaries, just as Dr. Amara has. By doing this, you
will be able to choose how you show up at work, at home,
and everywhere in between.

In these past few chapters, we've explored ideas to get
you started with creating boundaries. These boundaries can
focus on the following:

1. Fully disconnecting between work and home
2. Sharing the household workload and asking for help
3. Setting clear boundaries with people who drain
   your energy
4. Setting clear boundaries around how you handle
   money with others in your life
5. Creating a sacred physical and emotional space
   just for you

I'll see you in the last section of our book when you're ready to
take boundary-setting to the next level.

Reflection Questions

1. What important boundaries at home will you create?
2. How will these boundaries help you obtain freedom? What does freedom look like in your life? How will you know when you have it?
3. In these past few chapters, what topics have most resonated for you?
4. What changes do you need to make in your life to give yourself more space, time, and freedom?
5. Now that we have made it to this point of the book, what have you learned about yourself? How do you want your life to be different?
6. What do you commit to changing so you will have more freedom in your life?

WATCH VIDEO MESSAGE
FROM TAMMIE

PART V

CREATING THE LIFE YOU WANT

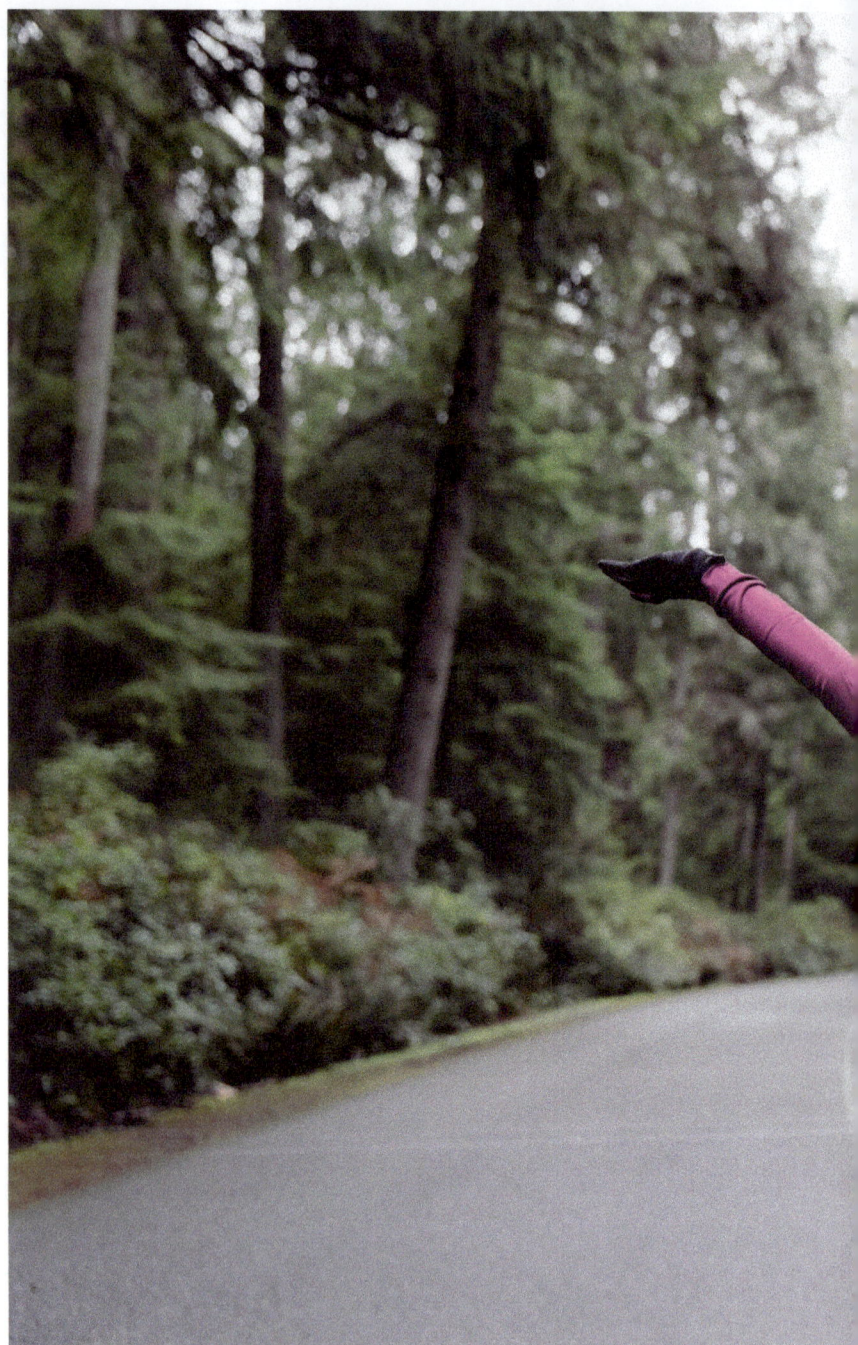

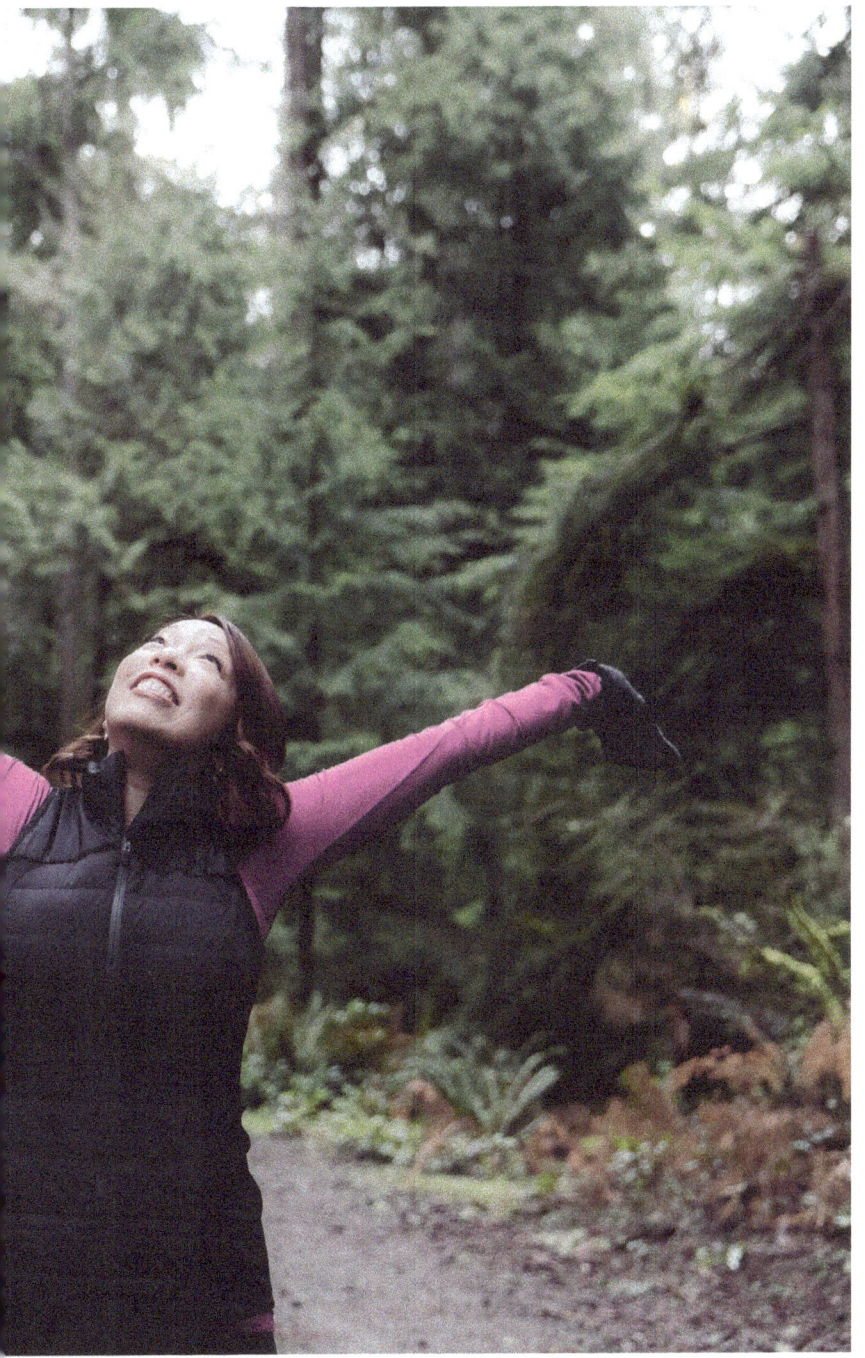

CHAPTER 20

CREATING THE
LIFE YOU WANT

So far in this book, we've walked through the lives of three awesome women physicians: Drs. Shruthi, Angela, and Amara. What all three women had in common at the beginning of their stories is a complete lack of boundaries, either within themselves, at work, or at home.

When we think about boundaries, we often think of them as being something we use to protect ourselves externally from other people. What I hope you've found through this book is that boundaries begin with you internally—from the inside out. Only when you have a clear understanding of yourself and what you need to be your best self, can you set definite boundaries to help you satisfy these needs. If you don't have this self-awareness, it will be very difficult to identify, establish, and maintain meaningful boundaries in either your professional or personal life.

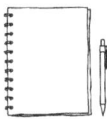

Key Concepts

Let's review some of the key concepts from this book:

1. **Boundaries start with you.** When we attain a clear sense of our values, our core purpose in life, our internal dialogue, our propensity for self-sabotage, and what we require to be our best selves—as represented by the metaphorical house discussed in Chapter 2—we can use this vision to create the boundaries necessary to sculpt all aspects of our lives.

2. **Boundaries at work.** As physicians, we have countless demands on our attention, energy, and time from patients, their families, staff, and colleagues. Plus, we must deal with the realities of being a doctor in today's healthcare world where administrative tasks, EMR, billing, and charting take up the bulk of our days. Setting clear boundaries in our work lives allows us to have control over all of these workplace elements and prevents them from taking over our lives. We must establish clear expectations to create the foundation for happy, healthy, and productive work relationships.

3. **Boundaries at home.** For most of us, our work doesn't end when we leave our jobs at the end of the workday because we have partners, children, family, friends, household, and financial responsibilities waiting for our attention at home, too. Sometimes this can make our home life seem like a second work shift. But by listening to your core values and using them to build healthy boundaries from the inside out, you can create a joyful life of freedom for yourself at home, too.

Weekly Time Log Exercise

How you spend your time is a very good indicator of what you value. There are 24 hours in a day and 168 hours in a week. Are you spending those hours in a way that is consistent with your core values? To find out, commit to doing this time log exercise for seven days. It will take some effort to complete but will be well worth it.

1. Refer to your workbook for the Weekly Time Log worksheet.
2. Use it to record everything you do each day of the week in 30-minute increments.
3. At the end of the week, tally up how much time you spend in each of these activities:
   a. Sleeping
   b. Eating
   c. Self-Care
   d. Commuting
   e. Working
   f. Emailing
   g. Charting & EMR
   h. Family time
   i. Watching TV
   j. Cell phone/social media use
   k. Other?
4. Reflect on whether the amount of time you spend doing each of these activities reflects your core values. Does it coincide with your Why and your personal impact statement?

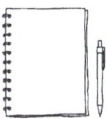

Ideal Week Exercise

Now that you've done the weekly time log exercise above, get ready to design your ideal week by completing this next exercise:

1. Refer to your workbook for the Ideal Week Exercise worksheet.

2. Using it, re-write the list of your weekly activities:
   a. Sleeping
   b. Eating
   c. Self-Care
   d. Commuting
   e. Working
   f. Emailing
   g. Charting & EMR
   h. Family time
   i. Watching TV
   j. Cell phone/social media use
   k. Other?

3. Now, next to each activity, record how many hours you want to spend each week doing each of them. This is a record of your Ideal Week.

4. Then write a comprehensive list of the boundaries you will institute both at work and at home that will allow you to spend your time each week doing what you want to do—in line with your core values. For example, these are my boundaries:
   a. No work email between 5:00 p.m. and 8:00 a.m. or on weekends

...continued overleaf

    b. Get seven to eight hours of sleep every night

    c. Meditate for five to ten minutes every morning before I get out of bed

    d. Exercise every day

    e. Spend quality time with my family every day

    f. Play the piano every day

5. Realize your boundaries don't need to be fancy or complicated. The simpler and clearer they are, the better. Try to attain them most days, understanding that unexpected issues arise and some of your boundaries may need to be adjusted. But you must first establish boundaries to attain results.

6. Post your completed Ideal Week Exercise somewhere you will see it every day.

Putting it All Together

Let's take a step back and look at the big picture. Recall the house metaphor we discussed at the beginning of the book, with the house as you, the fence as your boundaries, and the yard as the buffer between you and the outside world. Taking into consideration your Ideal Week Exercise, adjust your vision of each of these elements. What do your house, yard, and fence look like, now? How do you feel when you imagine being there?

Now, once again, picture yourself going up in a hot air balloon, way into the sky, and looking down on your metaphorical house. What do you see from that vantage point? Does the world you see align with your core values, your Why, and your purpose? How do you feel about yourself when you look below?

The chapters that follow will help you take this meta-view of your life and make it a reality.

Reflection Questions

1. What did you learn about yourself as you went through the Weekly Time Log and Ideal Week exercises?
2. How did your Weekly Time Log exercise compare with your core values, your Why, and your life goals?
3. When you took your second meta, hot-air balloon view of your house metaphor, how did it differ from your initial view at the beginning of the book?

CHAPTER 21

IDENTIFYING ENERGY ZAPPERS, ENERGY GIVERS, AND ENERGY MEHS

To be able to set clearly defined boundaries in our lives, we must build our self-awareness of what zaps our energy, what brings us energy, and what is neutral. I think of this neutral category as the "meh" category.

Initially, you may find it difficult to identify how your energy level is affected by different factors in your life, but I believe that deep down, we all have an inner wisdom that guides us in these matters if we allow ourselves to listen. Some call this our "gut instinct," others our "heart wisdom," and others still our "intuition." Regardless of the terminology, if we slow down and allow ourselves to notice how we are feeling in each moment, we can identify and access the space where our greatest power and freedom lives.

Let's do an exercise that will help you figure out what brings you energy, zaps your energy, or leaves it feeling meh.

Energy Awareness Exercise

Instructions:

1. Refer to your workbook for the Energy Awareness Exercise worksheet.
2. On this worksheet, brainstorm a list of every person and activity that demands your time and energy in each area of your life: self, work, and home. Include everyone you encounter and everything you do from when you wake up until you go to sleep at night. This includes a list of your family, friends, co-workers, and staff as well as basic hygiene tasks like showering and putting on makeup; home chores such as vacuuming, cleaning toilets, and washing the dishes; childcare responsibilities; work duties; emailing; driving ... Everything!
3. In the columns to the right of the worksheet, note whether each item zaps your energy, gives you energy, or is meh—neutral.
4. Now, fill in these lists: **My Energy Zappers, My Energy Givers, and My Energy Mehs.**
5. Read through the next few pages of this book in which we discuss what qualifies as your energy zappers, energy givers, and energy mehs. Then come back to complete steps 6 and 7 of this exercise.
6. Brainstorm what boundaries could be needed to address the Energy Zappers on your My Energy Zapper List. Notice how you feel as you go through this list. Notice when you feel tension as you write down your needed boundaries.

7. Brainstorm what boundaries could be needed to address the Energy Mehs on your My Energy Mehs list. Notice how you feel as you go through this list, and any tension as you write down your needed boundaries.

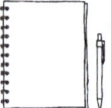

Your Energy Zappers

As you think about the items on your energy zapper list, notice how you feel in your arms, legs, belly, chest, and head. These physical symptoms caused by your energy zappers warn you that you are contemplating a person or situation that you dread dealing with. When you experience them, be aware, and consciously decide if you want to continue with that energy-zapping experience.

Numerous things in my life drain my energy. I enjoy video chats and virtual meetings for short periods, but they become energy zappers after several hours straight. When that happens, I feel like a zombie and know that I'm not even close to being my best self. Another zapper for me is a full day of back-to-back clinic patient appointments. I find I need to walk outside the building for a few minutes between appointments—even in the pouring rain—to breathe fresh air, clear my head, and regain my energy.

One of the most important lessons I learned in my adult life is that some people are energy zappers, and we need to limit our exposure to them. These may be people whose view of the world is negative, who espouse a victim mindset, who refuse to change, who are overly optimistic, or who are too needy. Maybe they are highly emotional and create too much drama around them. Only you know who triggers you emotionally and drains you. To conserve your energy, consider avoiding these people.

In the list you've made about the items that zap your energy, what boundaries have you've identified to counteract their effects? Examples might include rules like these:

1. Limit interaction at work with a draining colleague.
2. Mute text message and phone call alerts from people in your life who zap your energy or trigger you emotionally.
3. Remove work email and your EMR app from your phone so you're not tempted to check it at night or on weekends.
4. Remove social media from your phone, if you find it drains your energy or makes you feel bad about yourself.

Although you may find it difficult to set these boundaries, consider what your life will be like when these energy zappers are no longer present.

Your Energy Mehs

Now it's time to examine the items on your meh list, which are relatively neutral energy-wise. They won't zap your energy, but don't give you any either. This category often includes things you feel you should or are supposed to do—where your sense of obligation lies—and you often feel guilty if you say "no." When thinking about your meh items, you may not have a feeling of total dread, as with those on your energy zapper list, but your mehs don't bring you joy either.

My energy mehs include items like housework, yard work, shopping for groceries, picking up dry cleaning, and going to the post office. Writing chart notes and answering emails fall into this category, too, as do returning phone calls, completing prescription refills, and responding to in-basket messages. They're necessary, but not my favorite things to do.

Think about the items in your meh category and imagine what your life would be like if you could eliminate some of them. For many of these items, there may be no way to get rid of them completely, but you have other options like these:

1. Set a boundary that limits the meh's frequency or effect. Examples could include:
    a. Hire a laundry service, grocery delivery service, or house cleaners so that you delegate this responsibility to someone else.
    b. Only chart or answer email during designated times.
    c. Reserve evenings for wind-down time at home. No laptop, cell phone, or tablet use after a certain time in the evening.

2. Change your mindset about the item. (See sthe following uggestions on how to do this.)
3. Continue to feel meh about it.

As your coach and your friend, I challenge you to choose Option 1 or 2 to actively find a solution to your meh problems. I know you can do it!

Changing Your Mindset

In Chapter 8, we explored the cognitive behavioral therapy model of emotion. Now, let's use it to change your mindset about some of your energy mehs by altering your internal experience of each situation, stimuli, or person; the emotion you feel; and, ultimately, your behavior and the consequences of your behavior.

To see how this works, let's look at one of the items on my meh list: folding laundry. I do it because it needs to be done, and I'm picky about how I want my clothing folded, but I don't love it or even like it. Using the cognitive behavioral therapy model, instead of thinking, "Ugh, I have to fold laundry again," I say to myself, "While I fold laundry, I'll listen to my favorite podcast. It will be peaceful, and I'll learn something, too." Then I imagine how I will feel once all that laundry is nicely folded and put away. Ahhhh, what a relaxing thought! So, by using the cognitive behavioral therapy model, I took, "I have to fold the laundry," and turned it into, "I get to relax and listen to my favorite podcast while I fold my laundry, and then I won't have a huge pile of unfolded clothes on the top of my dryer weighing on my anymore. Awesome!" I no longer dread this task, but instead, look forward to it. My dread has transformed to enjoyment, maybe even a bit of joy.

I now challenge you to go through each item on your meh list and do the same thing. Consider your current mindset about each item and figure out an alternative, more enjoyable mindset to foster. Changing your mindset can significantly alter your experience of these tasks. They become less onerous and more neutral—maybe even a little bit enjoyable. Try it.

Your Energy Givers: How to Find Flow

Ah, we're finally talking about your energy givers—the items you want to do that allow you to be in a state of flow. "Flow," defined by psychologist Mihaly Csikszentmihalyi in *Flow: The Psychology of Optimal Experience* (Harper Perennial, 1990), is the state in which we are so absorbed in a situation or task that time passes by rapidly without us noticing. This is the experience of elite athletes, musicians, artists, mathematicians, scientists, and writers, who are most creative and most productive when they are in a state of flow. Stop and think of times in your life when you have found yourself in this condition of ease and focus, enjoying whatever you are doing.

What's even more wonderful about being in flow is that we not only feel fully absorbed at the moment but also often experience a rush of increased energy after completing the tasks. This energy often persists for several hours, or even days, afterward.

We set ourselves up to be in an optimal state of flow when we participate in activities and situations that are aligned with our core purpose and our core values. These energy-giving experiences allow us to be our most authentic selves and feel most alive.

Reflection Questions

1. Which of your energy zappers and meh items do you want to tackle first? How will you set boundaries and/or change your mindset about each of them?
2. Now consider the remaining items on your energy zapper and energy meh lists. How will you set boundaries and/or change your mindset about each one?
3. Look at your energy givers list. Of these items, which gives you the most flow? How can you increase your experience of flow with each item on this list?

CHAPTER 22

IDENTIFYING YOUR TEAM

A Team of Co-Workers, Friends, and Family

None of us is completely isolated. Even if we live alone, we still are blessed with close or extended family members, neighbors, friends, and co-workers. And when we begin to make changes in our lives—such as those suggested in this book—these people will be affected. As we explored in the Work and Home sections of the book, we saw that when we set new rules or boundaries for ourselves, the results may be uncomfortable for the people around us. They may feel confused and wonder what's wrong with you when you choose to live your life with intentionality you've never exhibited before.

When I coach women physicians, I walk them through scenarios they may experience with friends, family, and co-workers when they set boundaries from the inside out. We may discuss setting new expectations with a team member at their work or adhering to boundaries with their children. In all situations, the goal is to guide the doctors to help their co-workers, family, and friends understand their new boundaries so they, in turn, can assist the women in sustaining these boundaries. Alone, we can't affect these major changes in our lives, and it's almost universally better when we don't even try to do it by ourselves; we need a team.

An Opportunity for Deeper Connection

When asking others to help you make big changes in your life, such as the ones proposed in this book, let them know why these changes are important to you. My hunch is that many of your reasons relate to your core values and your Why. Share these reasons you want to change with the most trusted people in your life who you want as your allies in this work. You could start with just one person—perhaps your partner, a parent, a trusted friend, or a colleague at work. Connect with empathy, vulnerability, and honesty, and tell this person the why behind your request for help. And don't forget to ask her what she needs from you since she's probably struggling with setting boundaries, too.

When you ask someone for help setting a boundary, it creates an opportunity for a deeper connection with her. View this as an opportunity to form a better relationship with each important person in your life.

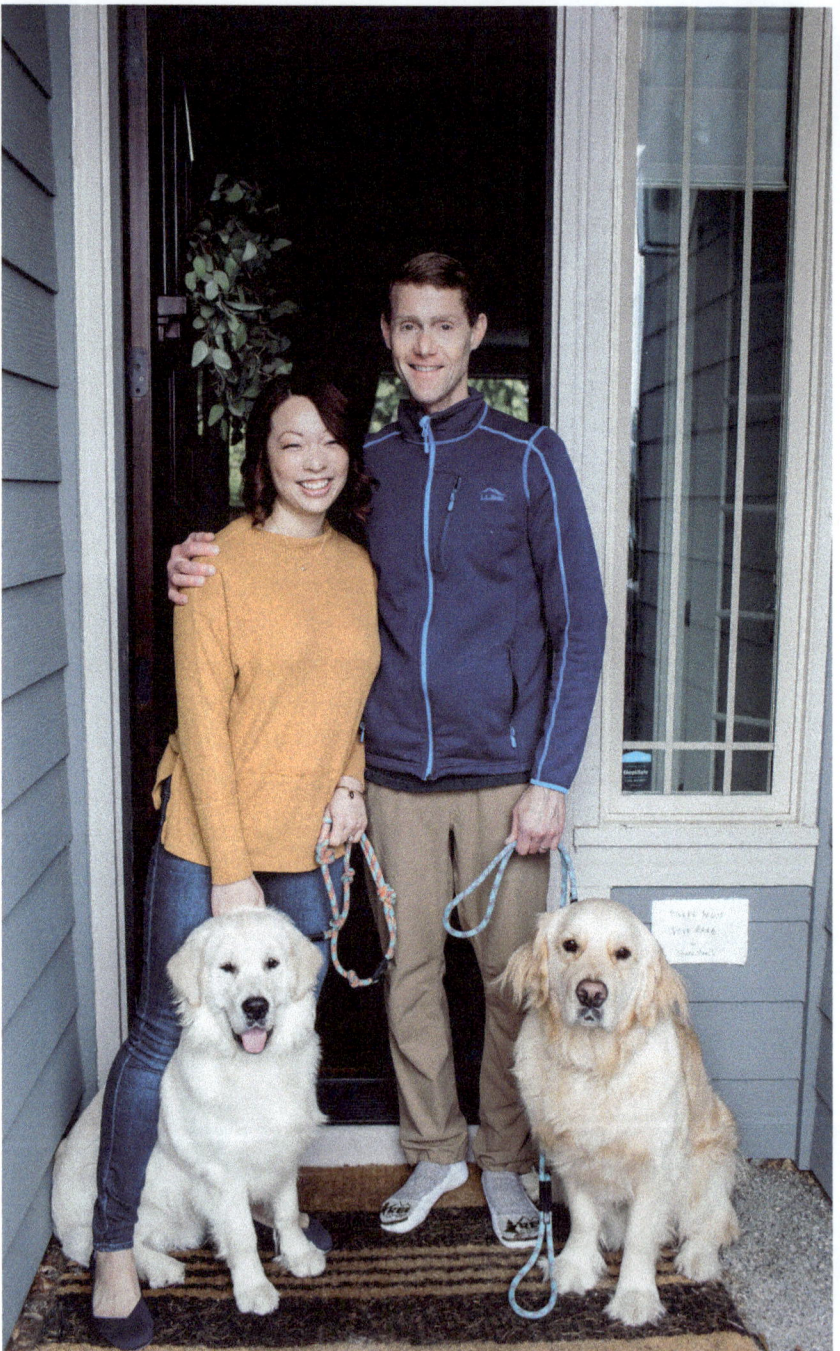

Exercise: Creating Your Team

Follow these steps to identify your personal boundary-setting teams:

1. Refer to your workbook for the Creating a Team to Fight My Top Three Energy Zappers worksheet.
2. Identify the three energy zappers you want to address first.
3. For each energy zapper, write down the rules or boundaries you will use to counteract them. Refer to your My Energy Zappers worksheet for the ideas you've brainstormed already.
4. Then answer these questions:
    a. Which people in my life will be most impacted by these new boundaries (specific co-workers, family members, and/or friends)?
    b. What does each person need to understand about my Why or my core values to help me implement my new boundaries? For example, you might say to your partner, "My top core values are joy, love, and freedom. To honor these core values, I need to prioritize our family more rather than working all the time."
    c. What expectations or ground rules do I need to set with each person for this item? An example might be that you ask your partner, "Will you please remind me at 7 p.m. each night that it is family time and I need to shut down my computer?"
    d. What personal behaviors do I need to commit

to, to ensure I remain strong and consistent with my new boundaries? For example, you commit to actually shutting down your computer and going downstairs to spend the evening with your family when your partner reminds you at 7 p.m.

e. What can I ask this person to do to help me maintain these behaviors? An example might be if you don't shut down your computer and come downstairs to relax with the family at 7 p.m., you give your partner permission to come upstairs and turn off your computer for you.

f. What personal boundaries does this person need to establish himself and how can I help him achieve them? For example, what does your partner need so that his core values and Why are in alignment?

5. Once you've finished your energy zapper worksheet, complete this one for your energy mehs: Creating a Team to Fight My Top Three Energy Mehs.

By completing these exercises, you have selected teams of people who you trust to help you combat your top energy zappers and energy mehs. Marvel at what you have just done for yourself. I'm so very proud of you!

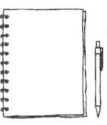

Your #1 Energy Zapper

Identifying the people who can help you deal with three of your energy zappers and three of your energy mehs is a very big first step toward instituting the boundaries necessary to create the life you long to have. However, making changes that affect six different problems may feel overwhelming to you. As a coach, one of my favorite questions to ask is, "What is the first step you need to take to make this change happen?" Think one baby step at a time.

So, let's get even more focused on setting your boundaries by looking at just one issue: your #1 energy zapper. In the worksheet in your Workbook, answer the following question:

1. What is your #1 energy zapper?
2. What rules or boundaries can your implement to counteract this zapper?
3. Who can help you accomplish these goals?
4. How can this person help you?
5. What first action will you take today to begin to deal with this #1 energy zapper?

Congratulations! You have just created a plan to set and implement your first boundary.

Not Just a Baby Step

I know working on your #1 energy zapper is only the first step in creating the many boundaries that will greatly improve your life. However, it's not just a baby step; it's huge, especially if you are the type of person who has previously struggled with setting healthy boundaries in your life. Being able to clearly state what you need and ask for help to obtain these needs are critical and essential steps toward change. Now comes the ongoing work of continuing this work, one new boundary at a time.

Reflection Questions

1. After reading this chapter what have you learned about yourself?
2. What have you learned about your relationships with the people in your life?
3. As you strive to set clear, consistent, and healthy boundaries for yourself, who will be your allies?
4. How does having a plan to deal with your #1 energy zapper make you feel?

CHAPTER 23

YOUR WHOLE-LIFE BOUNDARY PLAN

Putting All of the Pieces Together

In this book, we've touched on concepts and changes related to the different areas of your life, from your inner thoughts to your life at work and home. Give these new ideas time to sink in. Don't put too much pressure on yourself to adopt all of the concepts and strategies completely or immediately. I know as a woman physician, you try to get things done to the best of your abilities as soon as you possibly can. But change of this magnitude is going take time and daily practice. As the saying goes, "It's a marathon, not a sprint." Those of you who have run a marathon know that it takes weeks of consistent training to get you across that finish line on race day. No one in her right mind would try to run a marathon on Day Two after completing just one day of exercise.

Simply enacting your strategy for dealing with your #1 energy zapper may take weeks, months, or even years. It's a process, and it

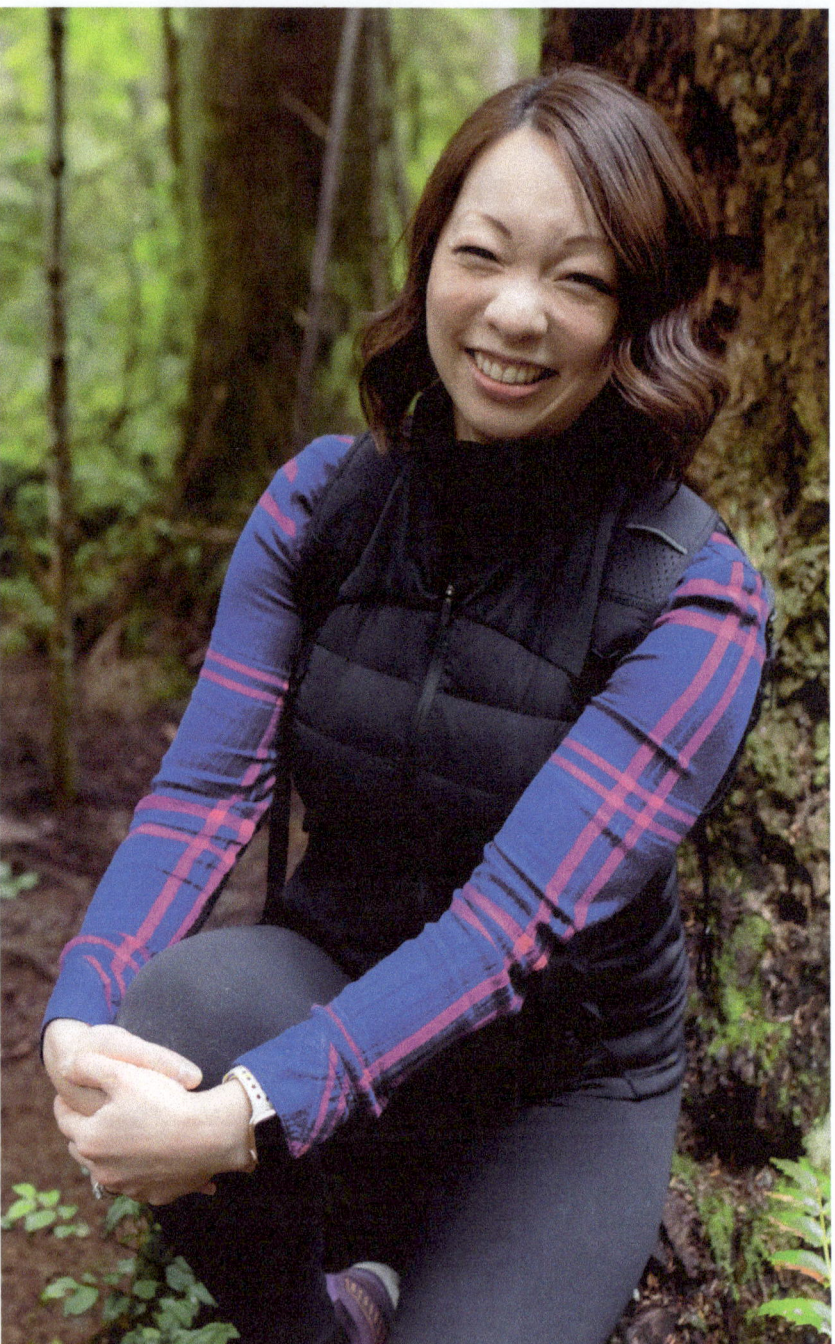

won't happen overnight. But know this: If you commit to working each day to implement the concepts from this book, and enlist your selected team to help you, you will succeed. For you, boundaries will become second nature.

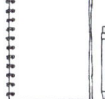

Exercise:
Creating Your Whole-Life
Boundary Plan

Once you've executed your plan for counteracting your #1 energy zapper and are ready to establish your next boundaries, review Chapters 21 and 22 and look at your lists of energy zappers, energy givers, and energy mehs. Then complete these steps to identify the next layer of changes you want to make in your life:

1. Refer to your workbook for the Your Whole Life Boundary Plan worksheet.
2. Refer to the chapters of this book that focused on establishing boundaries with yourself, at work, and at home.
3. Beginning with the worksheets on energy zappers and energy mehs you used to create your boundary-setting teams, make a list of the top three rules and boundaries you would like to establish in each area of your life:
   a. Self and Self-Care
   b. Work
   c. Home

4. For each of your proposed boundaries, select which of your team members will be ideally suited to help you establish and sustain it.
5. Identify and write down a concrete first step to making each of your boundaries a reality.

I know this may seem slightly overwhelming, but writing it all down is the most important step to make this a reality. Understand that this is merely the beginning of your marathon—the equivalent of being on Week Two of your training program. You've identified the necessary tools and learned how to use them. Now you must put them into practice every single day. It's okay to feel overwhelmed by the enormity of this task. This is why I'm here with you, even after you've finished reading this book. You can always ask yourself, "What Would Tammie Say?" Imagine me on your shoulder, guiding you as you strive to take each of these baby steps that will add up to big changes. Don't forget that you deserve a life and a career as a woman physician that you love and that brings you joy.

Reflection Questions

1. What one word describes how you feel about your Whole-Life Boundary Plan?
2. When you first started reading this book, what one word described how you were feeling about your personal boundaries?
3. What has been the most important lesson that you learned from this book?
4. What advice from this book would you give a friend?

CHAPTER 24

CONCLUSION:
LIVE YOUR VISION AND
BRING IT TO THE WORLD

**WATCH VIDEO
MESSAGE
FROM TAMMIE**

If you continue living as the woman physician you are today, what will you be like ten years from now? Will you be happy, joyful, full of life, and thriving? Or will you be exhausted, burned out, and feeling older than your years? What was it that compelled you to buy and read this book? Perhaps you feared looking into the future, only to see the image of a tired woman who looks beaten down by life and burdened with the needs of everyone around her.

Visualizing Your Future Life

I invite you to envision the life you would love to have in your wildest dreams. Don't hold back. Read this next paragraph, then close your eyes and visualize yourself in this life:

> Imagine yourself, ten years from now. You have done all the inner work mentioned in this book, and have set your clear expectations, goals, and boundaries. You are strong, calm, and centered. You feel energized and excited about your life. You find your work to be enjoyable. You are happy at home, too, and you feel connected to the people you care most about. In all aspects of your life, you are living your core values and your purpose. You are in flow, like a gentle stream traveling through a forest, feeling good about your life and where you are heading.

How does this meditation make you feel? What changes do you need to make for your dream life to become true? Here are some ways to get them started.

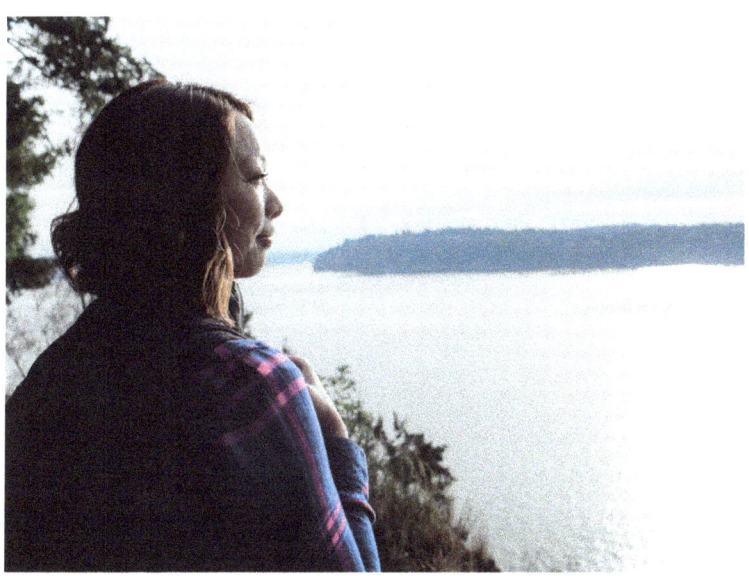

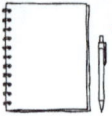

Dream Life Brainstorm

In your Workbook, write a list of everything you want to be true in your life. Only you can know what this means for you. Here are some examples to get you started:

- I love my life.
- Going to work is fun.
- I have energy at the end of my workday.
- I never have medical charts or work to do after work.
- When I go home, I love being there. My home life doesn't stress me out.
- I feel excited and energized about my goals and I am moving toward accomplishing the impact I want my life to have.
- I am healthy, strong, and in the best shape of my life physically, mentally, and emotionally.
- I spend quality time with the important people in my life, and I feel connected to my friends and family.
- I don't associate with people or situations that drain my energy.
- I do things because I choose to, not because I feel guilty or obligated.

Continue writing everything else you can think of that you want to be true in your life.

Choosing the Life You Lead

Remember that you get to consciously choose the life you want to have. But making a better life for yourself will not be easy. You must work hard to create a fulfilling life through self-reflection and self-realization followed by deliberate intention and actions, day after day, week after week, month after month, and year after year. You must push back against some of the lessons extolling self-sacrifice taught to you by your family, culture, and the medical establishment by setting boundaries, so you no longer give of yourself until you have nothing left.

Initially, you might find setting boundaries to be very difficult. Change is always uncomfortable. But when you feel this discomfort due to creating a new and better way of doing things, be assured you are on the right track, because it indicates you are living your life on purpose.

I want you to take an honest look at yourself right now. How well are the various areas of your life—self, work, and home—aligned to your core values, purpose, personal mission, and who you want to be in the world? How well do you set appropriate boundaries? Are you saying "yes" to the things that bring you joy and energy, and "no" to those that do not?

Now imagine what your life could be like if you fully aligned yourself with your core values. Who would you be? What kind of impact could you have on your community, the medical profession, and our world? Remember that when you live your most authentic self, you gain significant power.

My Closing Wish For You

My closing wish for you is that you go forth and be the change you want to see in the world. By putting the concepts in this book into practice every day with intention, you can become the woman and physician you long to be. Recognize that you have the power to choose the life you lead. Begin by caring for yourself and setting the limits and boundaries you need to become the very best version of your most authentic self. Dear friend, if you do this, you will inspire those around you to do the same. And the ripple effects will be endless.

I so believe in you. You've got this!

**WATCH CLOSING
VIDEO MESSAGE
FROM TAMMIE**

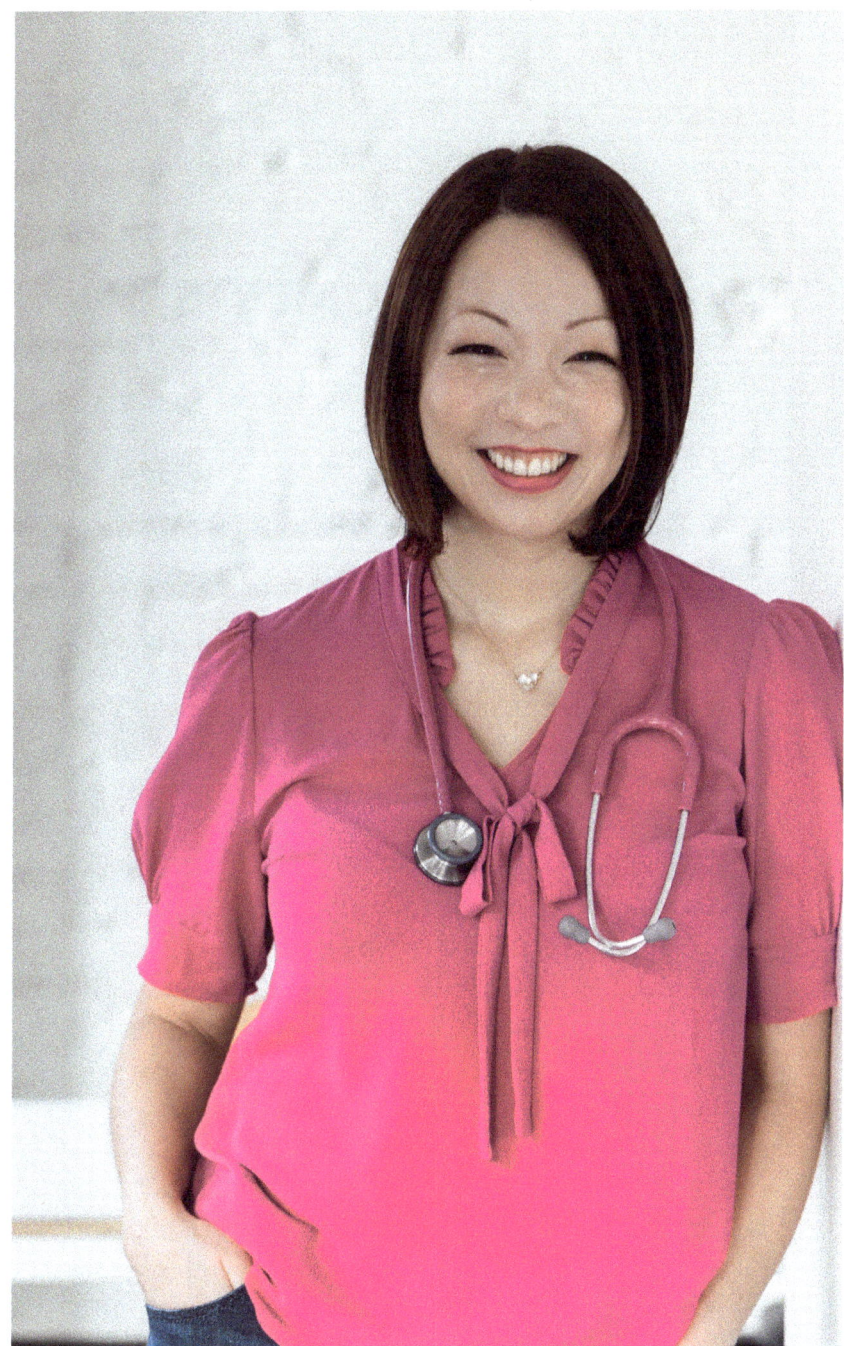

ACKNOWLEDGMENTS

This book was made possible through the support and assistance of many, to whom I am so very grateful.

First of all, I thank the most important person in my life, my husband, Matthew, who is my biggest supporter. I love you and our fur babies more than words can ever express.

And thank you to my parents, Kuo and Helen, my Papa and Mommy, who have shown me what true unconditional love is.

I am grateful to my dearest friends, Ross, Rachael, Luisa and Jen, who supported me at my lowest point. I love you and will be forever grateful to you for your love, compassion, and unconditional friendship.

My gratitude also goes out to my many other precious friends from each phase of my life. You know who you are. You have shown me what true friendship is.

And thank you to my teachers, mentors, coaches, and colleagues. You have taught me the true meaning of compassion, and of living a life in the service of others.

I also thank the people who contributed to crafting this book: Lynne Heinzmann, my editor, who expertly sculpted my rough draft into the polished work you now hold in your hands; Tamara Monosoff, my brilliant publisher who guided me through this entire process from start to finish; Marie O'Shepherd, my incredibly wonderful and talented book cover and interior designer who brought this book to life; Lisa Tener, my book coach, who introduced me to this whole new world of writing; Laura Pasquale, my copyeditor and proofreader, for whom I am so incredibly grateful; Dan Thibeault of Fast Twitch Media, who expertly edited all of the videos created for this book; my publicity team at Zilker Media who expertly guided me through this new world of public media; Jamie Palmer, my business coach, and Outlier Marketing Group for helping me share my message through the power of social media; and finally, Jennifer Kimpe, my dear friend and talented brand strategist, who helped me to take this book from a simple idea to reality, and to Sophia Mavrides, whose stunning photography and talent for design has brought this entire project to life.

ABOUT THE AUTHOR

Tammie Chang, MD

Dr. Tammie Chang is a board-certified physician in pediatric hematology/oncology practicing in Tacoma, Washington. She is also a certified leadership coach for women physicians and the Co-Founder of Pink Coat, MD, a digital platform to support women physicians in their careers and in living their best lives (www.pinkcoatmd.com). Together with Dr. Luisa Duran, Tammie co-authored the Amazon bestselling book, *How to Thrive as a Woman Physician* (Pink Coat, MD; 2021).

Tammie is the Medical Director of her health system's Provider Wellness Program and Founder and Director of her hospital's Pediatric Cancer Survivorship Program. In addition, she serves as the Washington State Physician Branch President of the American Medical Women's Association (AMWA) and the Program Director of ELEVATE,

AMWA's National Leadership Development Program for Women Physician Attendings.

Tammie earned her bachelor's degree and medical degree from Brown University and completed her combined internal medicine and pediatrics residency at the University of Massachusetts. She completed her fellowship in pediatric hematology/oncology at St. Jude Children's Research Hospital.

Tammie received leadership coaching certifications from the Co-Active Training Institute and the International Coaching Federation. She is also certified as a John Maxwell Leadership Coach, Trainer, and Speaker; a Gallup CliftonStrengths Coach; and a Tara Mohr Playing Big Facilitator.

Tammie lives in the Pacific Northwest with her husband, Matthew, and their four fur babies: Golden retrievers, Gus and Toby, and cats, Ellie and Mimi. The favorite moments of her day involve playing Rachmaninoff and Chopin on the piano and being active in the beautiful outdoors with her family. To contact Tammie or learn more about her coaching programs, visit her website at www.tammiechangmd.com.

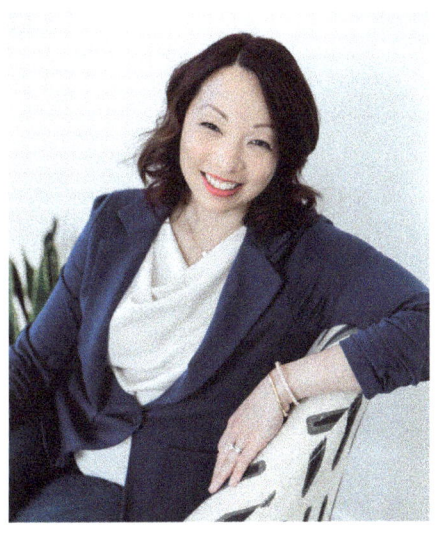

REFERENCES

PART I

Chapter 1

Collier, R. (2018). Addressing physician burnout at the systems level. *CMAJ, 190*(6): E174.

Farmer, B. (Host) (July 31, 2018). When doctors struggle with suicide, their profession often fails them [Audio podcast episode]. In Shots: *Health News from NPR*. NPR. https://www.npr.org/sections/health-shots/2018/07/31/634217947/to-prevent-doctor-suicides-medical-industry-rethinks-how-doctors-work

Hampton, T. (September 14, 2005). Experts address the risk of physician suicide. *Journal of American Medical Association, 294*(10), 1189-91. DOI: 10.1001/jama.294.10.1189.

Menon, N.K., Shanafelt T.D. et al. (December 2020). Association of physician burnout with suicidal ideation and medical errors. *Journal of American Medical Association, 3*(12):e202870. DOI: 10.1001/jamanetworkopen.2020.28780.

Paturel, A. (October 1, 2019). *Why women leave medicine* [Press release]. Retrieved from https://www.aamc.org/news-insights/why-women-leave-medicine

Schernhammer, E.S., & Colditz, G.A. (December 2004). Suicide rates among physicians: a quantitative and gender assessment (meta-analysis). *American Journal of Psychiatry, 161*(12):2295-302. DOI: 10.1176/appi. ajp.161.12.2295

The Physicians Foundation (2012). *A Survey of America's Physicians: Practice Patterns and Perspectives,* Author.

West, C.P., Dyrbye, L.N., & Shanafelt, T.D. (2018). Physician burnout: contributors, consequences, and solutions. *Journal of Internal Medicine, 283*(6), 516-569. DOI: 10.1111/joim.12752

Chapter 2

Cloud, H., Townsend, J. *Boundaries: When to say yes, how to say no.* Thomas Nelson Publishing, 1992.

Johnson, R. *Setting boundaries and setting limits.* BPDFamily, 2014.

Merriam-Webster.com. Definition of '"metaphor."

Nagoski A., Nagoski, E. *Burnout: the secret to unlocking the stress cycle.* Ballantine Books, 2020.

PART II

Chapter 4

Brown, B. *Dare to Lead: Brave Work. Tough Conversations. Whole Hearts.* Penguin Random House, 2018.

Sinek, S. *Start with Why: How Great Leaders Inspire Everyone to Take Action.* Portfolio, 2011.

Chapter 5

Brown, B. *Dare to Lead: Brave Work. Tough Conversations. Whole Hearts.* Penguin Random House, 2018.

Neff, K. D. (2012). The science of self-compassion. In C. Germer & R. Siegel (Eds.), *Compassion and Wisdom in Psychotherapy* (pp.79-92). New York: Guilford Press.

Chapter 6

Adolphs, R. (Jan 2013). The biology of fear. *Current Biology: 23*(2): R79-R93.

Day, A.L., Caroll, S.A. (April 2004). Using an ability-based measure of emotional intelligence to predict individual performance, group performance, and group citizenship behaviors. *Personality and Individual Differences, 36*(6):1443-145, doi:10.1016/@0191-8869(03)00240-X

Dutheil F et al. (Dec 2019). Suicide among physicians and health-care workers: a systematic review and metaanalysis. *PLoS ONE, 14*(12):e0226361, doi:10.1371/journal.pone.0226361

Houkes, I, Winants, Y et al (April 2011). Development of burnout over time and the causal order of the three dimensions of burnout among male and female GPs. A three-wave panel study. *BMC Public Health* 11, 240, doi:10.1186/1471-2458-11-240

Melnick, EF, Ong SY et al (May 2021). Characterizing physician HER use with vendor-derived data: a feasibility study and cross-sectional analysis. *Journal of the American Medical Informatics Association, 28*(7):1383-1392, doi:10.1093/jamia/ocab011

Tswgawa, Y; Jena, A.B. et al (February 2017). Comparison of hospital mortality and readmission rates for Medicare patients treated by male vs female physicians. *Journal of American Medical Association, 177*(2):206-213. doi:10.1001/jamainternmed.2016.7875

West, C.P., Dyrbye, L.N., Shanafelt, T.D. (March 2018). Physician burnout: contributors, consequences, and solutions. *Journal of Internal Medicine, 283*(6):516-529, doi:10.1111/joim.12752

Chapter 7

American College of Lifestyle Medicine https://www.lifestylemedicine.org/

Kalmbach, D.A. et al. (March, 2017). Sleep disturbance and short sleep as risk factors for depression and perceived medical errors in first-year residents. *Sleep*, 40(3):zsw073. doi:10.1093/sleep/zsw073

Trockel, M.T. et al. (December 2020). Assessment of physician sleep and wellness, burnout, and clinically significant medical errors. *Journal of American Medical Association*, *3*(12):e2028111, doi:10.1001/jamanetworkopen.2020.28111

PART III

Chapter 13

Paturel, A. (October 1, 2019). Why women leave medicine [Press release]. Retrieved from https://www.aamc.org/news-insights/why-women-leave-medicine

PART IV

Chapter 15

AAMC (December 2019). The majority of U.S. medical students are women, new data show. https://www.aamc.org/news-insights/press-releases/majority-us-medical-students-are-women-new-data-show

Canfield, J., Hansen, M., Hewitt, L. *The Power of Focus*. Vintage/Ebury, 2001.

Germano, M. (March 2019). Women are working more than ever, but they still take on most household responsibilities. Forbes.

Paturel, A. (October 2019). Why women leave medicine. *AAMC*. https://www.aamc.org/news-insights/why-women-leave-medicine

U.S. Bureau of Labor Statistics (December 2017). Percentage of employed women working full time little changed over last 5 decades. https://www.bls.gov/opub/ted/2017/percentage-of-employed-women-working-full-time-little-changed-over-past-5-decades.htm

U.S. Bureau of Labor Statistics (April 2021). Women in the labor force: a databook. https://www.bls.gov/opub/reports/womens-databook/2020/home.htm

Chapter 17

AAMC (February, 2021). Taking control of credit card debt. https://students-residents.aamc.org/financial-aid-resources/taking-control-credit-card-debt

Educationdata.org (July, 2021). Average medical school debt. https://educationdata.org/average-medical-school-debt

Medscape (August, 2020). Medscape residents salary and debt report 2020. https://www.medscape.com/slideshow/2020-residents-salary-debt-report-6013072

PART V

Chapter 21

Csikszentmihali, M. *Flow: the psychology of optimal experience*. Harper Perennial, 1990.

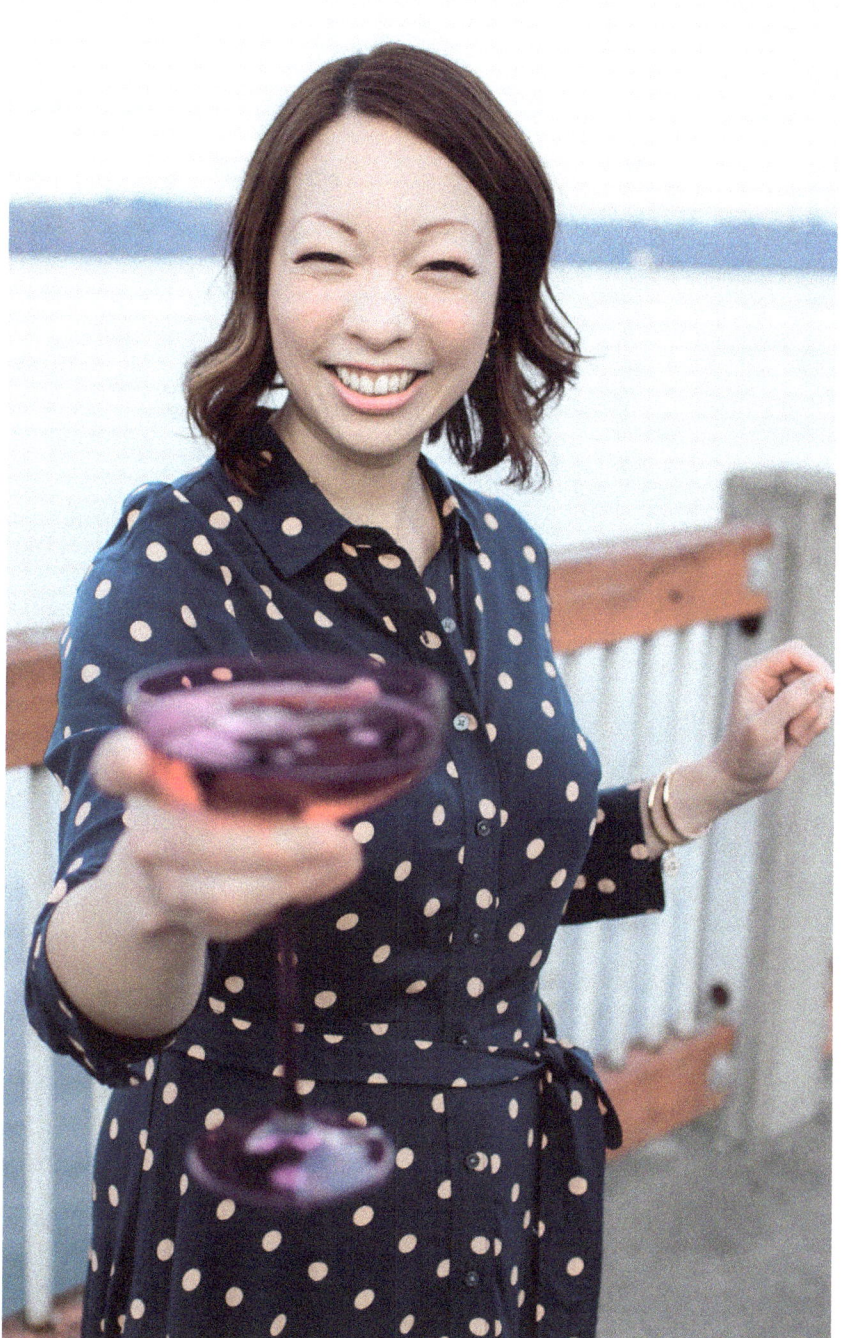

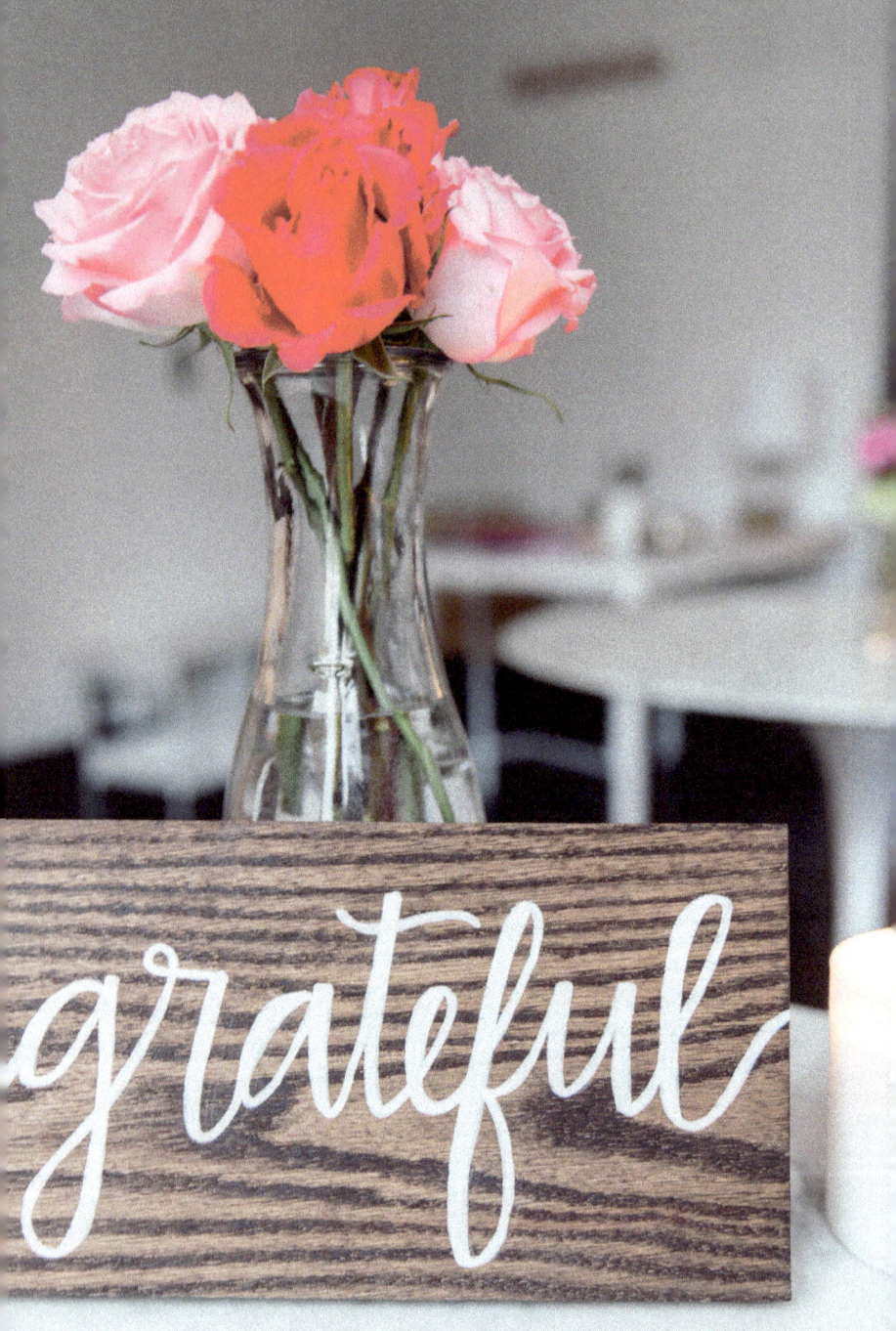